Langman's Essential Medical Embryology

Langman's Essential Medical Embryology

T. W. Sadler, PhD

Consultant, Embryology and Birth Defects Prevention
Twin Bridges
Madison County, Montana

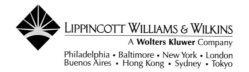

LIPPINCOTT WILLIAMS & WILKINS
A **Wolters Kluwer** Company

Philadelphia • Baltimore • New York • London
Buenos Aires • Hong Kong • Sydney • Tokyo

Acquisitions Editor: Betty Sun
Managing Editor: Sonya L. Seigafuse
Marketing Manager: Joe Schott
Production Editor: Caroline Define
Designer: Doug Smock
Compositor: TechBooks
Printer: R.R. Donnelley

To purchase additional copies of this book, call our customer service department at **(800) 638-3030** or fax orders to **(301) 824-7390**. International customers should call **(301) 714-2324**.

Visit Lippincott Williams & Wilkins on the Internet: http://www.LWW.com. Lippincott Williams & Wilkins customer service representatives are available from 8:30 am to 6:00 pm, EST.

05 06 07 08
2 3 4 5 6 7 8 9 10

To all students trying to learn embryology.

PREFACE

This first edition of *Langman's Essential Medical Embryology* represents the first truly "essentials" version of the topic that provides a concise but thorough description of embryology and its clinical significance. It is a unique combination of text and figures that, together, convey important concepts and an understanding of the subject. Also, included is *Simbryo,* an interactive CD-ROM that demonstrates normal embryological events and the origins of some birth defects. This unique program offers six original vector art animation modules that illustrate the complex, three-dimensional aspects of embryology. Together, *Langman's Essential Medical Embryology* and *Simbryo* provide the most comprehensive and understandable presentation of the subject in the most concise format available.

Langman's Essential Medical Embryology is a combination of concise text and figures that must be used together to gain comprehension of the subject. Figures have been grouped to better illustrate key points, which are explained succinctly. The artwork is extensive and includes 4-color line drawings and scanning electron micrographs. Each chapter also contains clinical material, including figures, to illustrate how important embryology is to understanding the origin, treatment, and prevention of birth defects. Also provided is an overview of the key genes involved in normal development and the origin of birth defects.

Embryology is a fascinating subject with relevance for many types of health care and public health officials. Serious birth defects occur in approximately 6% of children and are the leading cause of infant mortality. Thus, understanding embryology is the first step toward their prevention and treatment. Hopefully, you will find that *Langman's Essential Medical Embryology* makes the learning process simpler and easier than it has ever been.

T.W. Sadler
Twin Bridges, Montana

CONTENTS

CHAPTER 1

Introduction: Basic Principles of Development

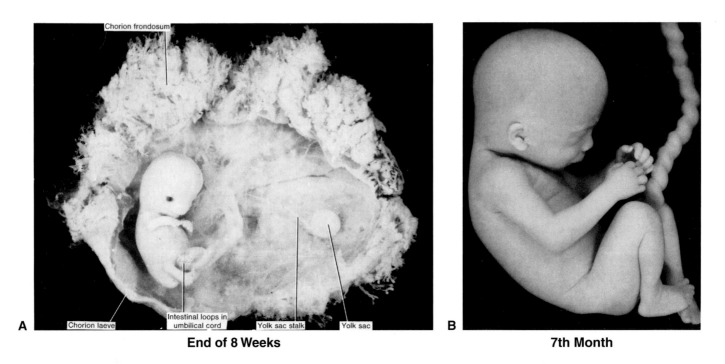

End of 8 Weeks   **7th Month**

FIGURE 1.1. **Embryology** is the study of development of an organism from fertilization of the ovum—the single cell stage—through the period of **organogenesis**, when primordia of the organ systems are established. In the human, this time frame encompasses the first **8 weeks** of pregnancy (**A**). At that point, the developing human enters the **fetal period**, when differentiation continues and weight and length are increased (**B**). At the end of 8 weeks, the embryo's **crown–rump length** (CRL), the measurement from the top of the head to the rump, is approximately 3 cm, and it weighs 8 to 10 g. At birth (38 weeks), the infant's CRL is 35 cm, and it weighs 3200 g. So how does an embryo progress from a single cell to nearly a complete organism in a period of 8 weeks? The process is complex but not daunting to understand, especially now that many of the molecular signals regulating development are being elucidated. Several cellular events are essential to the process: (1) Cell proliferation increases cell number in preparation for cell differentiation. Cell division (cycle) times in the embryo are as little as 4 hours, so there can be a 32-fold increase in cell number in a 24-hour period. Such short cell cycle times begin at very early stages but also occur in each organ system as that system initiates its development. These proliferative phases are highly sensitive to insult from genetic or environmental factors. Consequently, the embryo itself, followed by each organ system, passes through a stage when it is most sensitive to these insults. If such an insult occurs very early, the embryo usually dies; if it occurs later during organogenesis, then one or more organs may develop abnormally, resulting in one or more birth defects. (2) Cell migration occurs as cells move into position to create differentiated cell types. Once again, this is a vulnerable time for cells, and they may be affected directly or indirectly via the matrix through which they travel. (3) Cell differentiation is the completion of cell development, when cells assume their ultimate phenotype. As this process is initiated, cell proliferation decreases and cells become less vulnerable to insult.

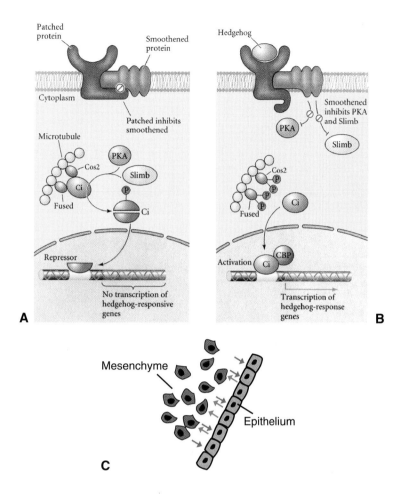

FIGURE 1.2. The molecular signals responsible for many of these cellular phenomena have been identified. For example, many genes regulating the cell cycle have been described and their roles determined. Likewise, regulatory genes for cell-to-cell communication as well as tissue interactions have been delineated. Regulation of these events invariably depends on genetic cascades involving signal molecules and their receptors, such as **growth factors** and **morphogens** together with **transcription factors** that code for DNA-binding proteins. These proteins bind to DNA and regulate expression of downstream genes. A classic example of such a signaling pathway, used repeatedly by embryos, involves the secreted morphogen *sonic hedgehog* (*SHH;* **A** and **B**). In the absence of *SHH,* its membrane receptor patched inhibits another protein called smoothened. Without smoothened activity, the cubitus interruptus (Ci) protein is bound to microtubules by Cos2 and fused proteins, where it is cleaved by protein kinase A (PKA) and slimb proteins. A cleaved portion of the Ci protein then binds to DNA and inhibits transcription of other genes (**A**). Once SHH arrives and binds to its receptor, patched, smoothened is activated, which, in turn, inactivates the Ci cleaving proteins PKA and slimb. As a result, Ci remains intact and is released from the microtubules when Cos2 and fused are inactivated by phosphorylation. Now Ci can bind to DNA and act as a transcriptional activator of **SHH** response genes (**B**). Note that this pathway is activated by inhibiting an inhibitor, another recurring theme during embryogenesis. Several families of growth factors and morphogens exist, including members of the WNT, transforming growth factor-β (TGF-β; includes nodal and BMPs), fibroblast growth factor (FGF), and SHH families. These families are large, with some including 15 or more members, which increases complexity but also provides many avenues and variations for regulatory control. During organogenesis, these factors regulate many developmental events, and one of the most common of these involves **epithelial-mesenchymal interactions** (**C**). Virtually all organ systems depend on this type of interaction to initiate their differentiation. From the eye, to the limb, to the gut, to the gonads, communication between epithelial and mesenchymal tissue types is essential. Molecular signals pass from one to the other using growth factors and morphogens as both types of tissues are instructed to differentiate into their definitive structures (**C**). This interaction is fundamental to embryonic development and represents another vulnerable target for disruption. The efficiency of the process of embryogenesis is not great, and sensitivity to genetic or environmental alteration is a real issue. In fact, over 50% of fertilized ova are aborted (most so early in development that a woman never realizes she has conceived), and, of those that are aborted, over 50% have chromosomal abnormalities. Furthermore, 4% to 6% of liveborn infants suffer from a serious structural defect, e.g., cleft palate or neural tube defect. Most of the insults occur during the first 8 weeks of gestation, when basic cell processes are taking place. When all of these processes culminate in a new healthy human being, however, the phenomenon of embryogenesis is an awesome event.

CHAPTER 2

Early Development: Fertilization to Gastrulation

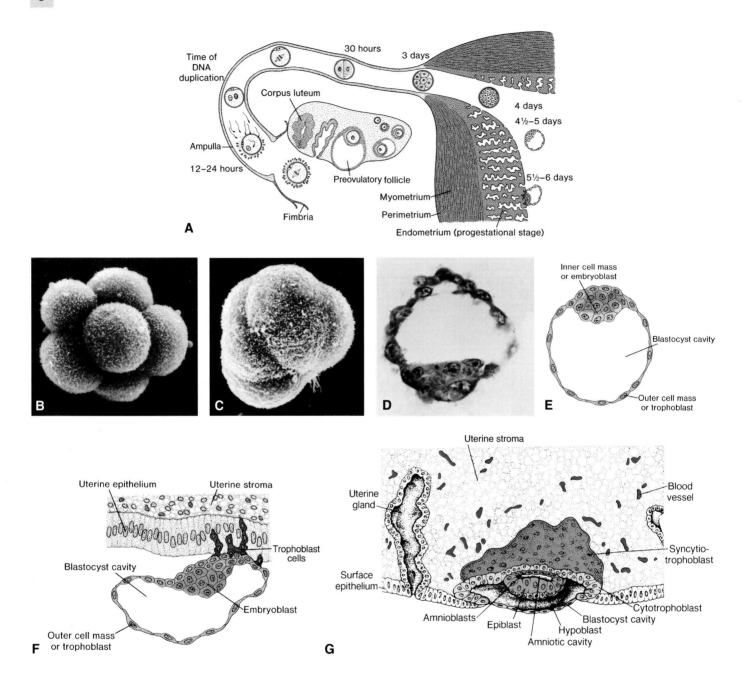

FIGURE 2.1. **Fertilization** (fusion of the sperm and egg) normally occurs in the ampullary region of the uterine (fallopian) tube within 24 hours of ovulation (**A**). Once the sperm enters the egg, the male and female pronuclei come into close contact and replicate their DNA, and cell division then occurs, creating a two-cell embryo. Cell division continues as the embryo proceeds along the uterine tube toward the uterus (**A**). Three days after fertilization, the embryo consists of a ball of cells called the **morula** (mulberry) and resides at the opening (os) of the uterine tube into the uterine cavity (**A** and **B**). At about this time, cells of the morula undergo **compaction**, a process whereby cell-to-cell contacts are maximized through tight junctions, and inner cells are segregated from outer cells (**C**). As subsequent cell divisions occur, a small group of inner cells (the **inner cell mass**, or **embryoblast**) becomes segregated from the outer cells (the **outer cell mass** or **trophoblast**). Over the next 2 days, fluid is pumped from the outside to the inside, and the morula is transformed into a hollow **blastocyst (D and E)**. The inner cell mass gives rise to the entire embryo and is displaced to one pole of the blastocyst, the embryonic pole; the outer cell mass forms the outer layer of the blastocyst and contributes to development of the placenta. About the sixth day, the blastocyst implants by attaching itself to the uterine epithelium and then, over the next several days, invades this tissue (**A** and **F**). By this time, the trophoblast has differentiated into two layers: an invasive outer multinucleated cytoplasmic mass called the **syncytiotrophoblast**, and an inner proliferative layer that provides additional trophoblast cells, the **cytotrophoblast** (**F** and **G**). **Implantation** occurs when syncytiotrophoblast overlying the embryonic pole interacts with uterine epithelial cells to promote adhesion, followed by invasion of the blastocyst (**F** and **G**).

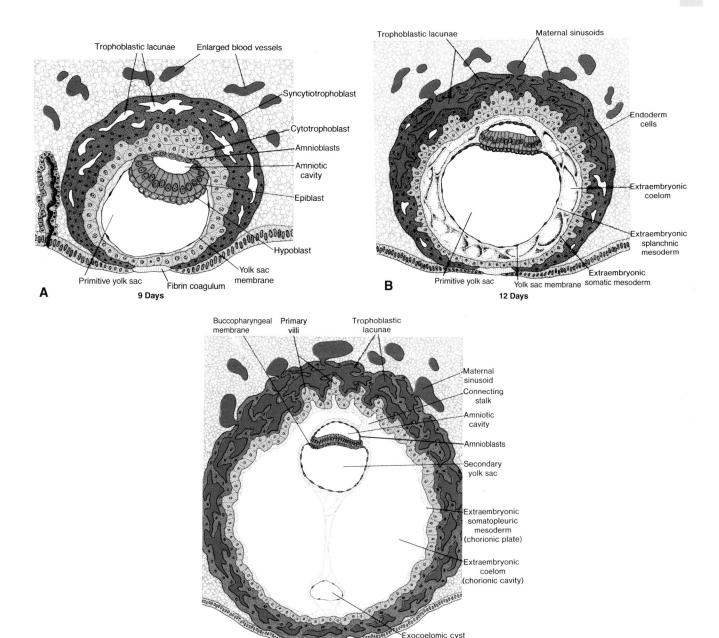

FIGURE 2.2. The second week of development is called the "week of twos." The trophoblast is differentiated into two layers, the **syncytioblast** and the **cytotrophoblast**; the **embryoblast** reorganizes into two layers, the **epiblast** dorsally and the **hypoblast** ventrally; two cavities are formed, the **amniotic cavity** dorsal to the epiblast and the **yolk sac cavity** ventral to the hypoblast; and two layers of extraembryonic mesoderm are formed between the embryo and its cavities and the cytotrophoblast (**A** and **B**). The epiblast and hypoblast appear as a slightly elongated disc (the **bilaminar germ disc**), like a cookie with no icing in the center, and it is the epiblast that will give rise to all of the tissues of the embryo. In addition, proliferation of epiblast cells at the margins of the disc forms amnioblasts that line the amniotic cavity. In a similar fashion, a primitive yolk sac is created by proliferation of hypoblast cells at the disc margins (**A**). Thus, the embryonic disc is suspended between these two cavities. Meanwhile, trophoblast cells continue to invade the uterine wall until the conceptus is surrounded by uterine tissue. By 12 to 14 days, cells of the syncytiotrophoblast erode uterine blood vessels, and maternal blood fills spaces (lacunae) that form in the syncytium, bringing nutrients closer to the developing embryo (**B** and **C**). In addition, **extraembryonic mesoderm** is formed by delamination of yolk sac cells and later by migration of cells through the primitive streak during gastrulation (**B** and **C**; Chapter 2; Fig. 2.4). Initially, this tissue forms as a single layer, but it soon separates into two layers: a layer around the yolk sac, which is the **extraembryonic splanchnic mesoderm**, and a layer over the amnion and on the inner surface of the cytotrophoblast, which is the **extraembryonic somatic mesoderm** (**C**). The two layers remain connected to each other at the **connecting stalk**, which will contribute to formation of the **umbilical cord** (**C**). The cavity between the layers is called the **extraembryonic cavity**. By the beginning of the third week, this cavity will be well defined and will form the **chorionic cavity**, while the somatic layer of extraembryonic mesoderm will form the **chorion**. This mesoderm also will form the core of the primary villi of the placenta.

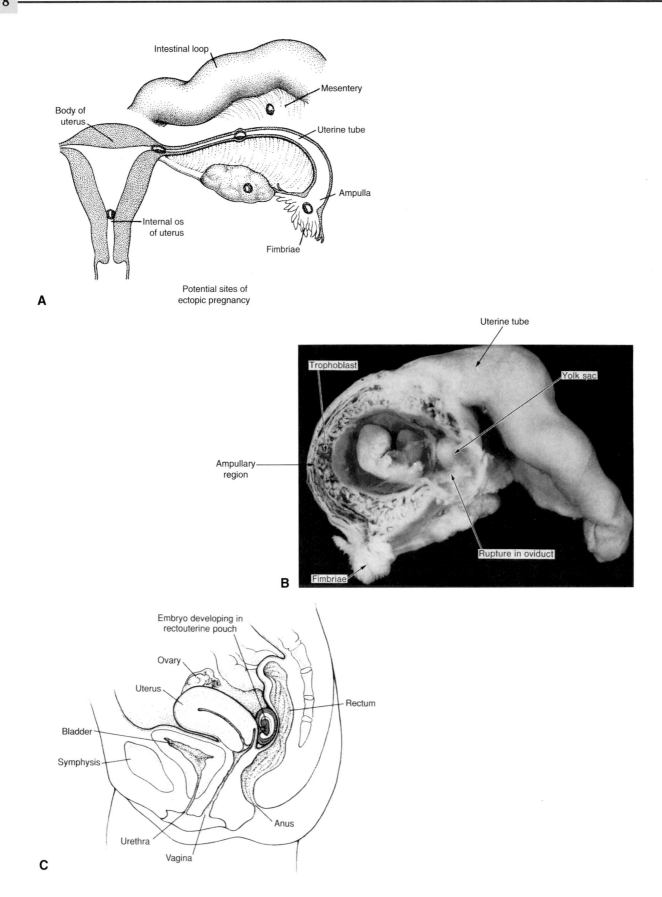

A

Intestinal loop

Mesentery

Body of
uterus

Uterine tube

Internal os
of uterus

Ampulla

Fimbriae

Potential sites of
ectopic pregnancy

B

Uterine tube

Trophoblast

Yolk sac

Ampullary
region

Rupture in oviduct

Fimbriae

C

Embryo developing in
rectouterine pouch

Ovary

Uterus

Rectum

Bladder

Symphysis

Anus

Urethra

Vagina

FIGURE 2.3.   Because of the invasive nature of the syncytiotrophoblast, blastocysts occasionally implant at sites outside the main body of the uterus (**A**). These **ectopic pregnancies** usually occur in the ampullary region of the uterine tube (**B**), but may occur in other areas as well, even in the peritoneal cavity. In this area the most likely site is in the rectouterine (Douglas') pouch, between the uterus and rectum (**C**). All ectopic pregnancies are dangerous because of the potential for the invasive tissue of the blastocyst to cause severe bleeding.

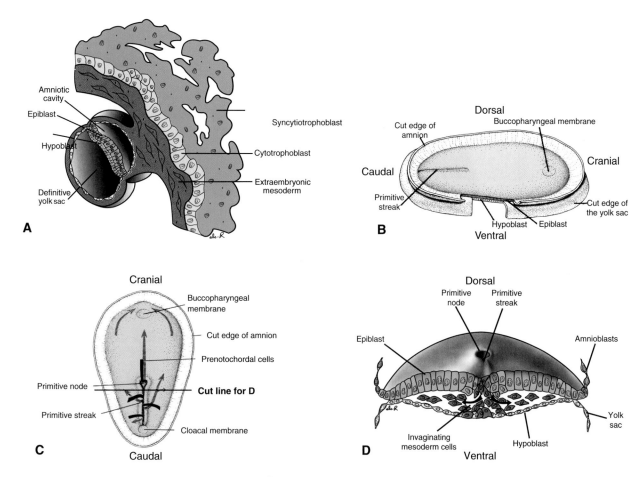

Table 2.1. **Derivatives of the Three Primary Germ Layers**

Germ Layer	Derivative
Ectoderm	Central nervous system
	Peripheral nervous system
	Epidermis, hair, nails
	Sensory epithelium: nose, ear, eye
Mesoderm	
Paraxial	Part of skull, muscles, vertebrae
Intermediate	Urogenital system
Lateral plate	
Visceral layer	Serous membranes around organs
Parietal layer	Serous membranes, body wall, limbs
Endoderm	Gut tube and its derivatives : glands, lungs, liver, gallbladder, pancreas

FIGURE 2.4. The third week is called the "week of threes." During this period, the bilaminar germ disc is transformed by the process of **gastrulation** into three germ layers: (1) **ectoderm**, which will form the central and peripheral nervous systems, the epidermis (including hair and nails), and sensory epithelia of the ear, nose, and eyes; (2) **mesoderm**, which will form muscle, bone, connective tissue, blood and blood vessels, serous membranes, and the urogenital system; and (3) **endoderm**, which will form the gut tube and all of its derivatives (glands, lungs, liver, gallbladder, and pancreas; Table 2.1. Three cavities will become defined: the **amniotic**, **yolk sac**, and **chorionic cavities** (Fig. 2.2C). At the same time, three layers will be established in the **placental villi**: the outer **syncytiotrophoblast**; the **chorionic mesoderm** on the inside; and the **cytotrophoblast** in the middle (Fig. 2.2C). **Gastrulation** is the process involving cell movements that transforms the bilaminar embryonic disc into a trilaminar structure comprised of the three primary germ layers of the embryo. It begins by formation of the **primitive streak** in the **epiblast** at the caudal end of the embryonic disc (**A** and **B**). This streak actually is a groove with a pit at its cranial end. Cells around the pit are elevated, and together the cells and pit form the **primitive node** (**C** and **D**). Once the streak and node are formed, epiblast cells migrate toward these structures and then turn into the streak and node, where they detach and continue their migration beneath the remaining epiblast (**C** and **D**). Some of these cells migrate ventrally and displace existing hypoblast cells to create a new layer, the endoderm (**D**). Others migrate between this new layer and the epiblast to form a middle layer, the mesoderm—the "icing" in the cookie (**D**). Thus, three embryonic germ layers are established: those cells remaining in the epiblast form ectoderm; those that migrate and displace the hypoblast form endoderm; and those that migrate to the middle layer form mesoderm. Note that all three layers are derived from the original epiblast.

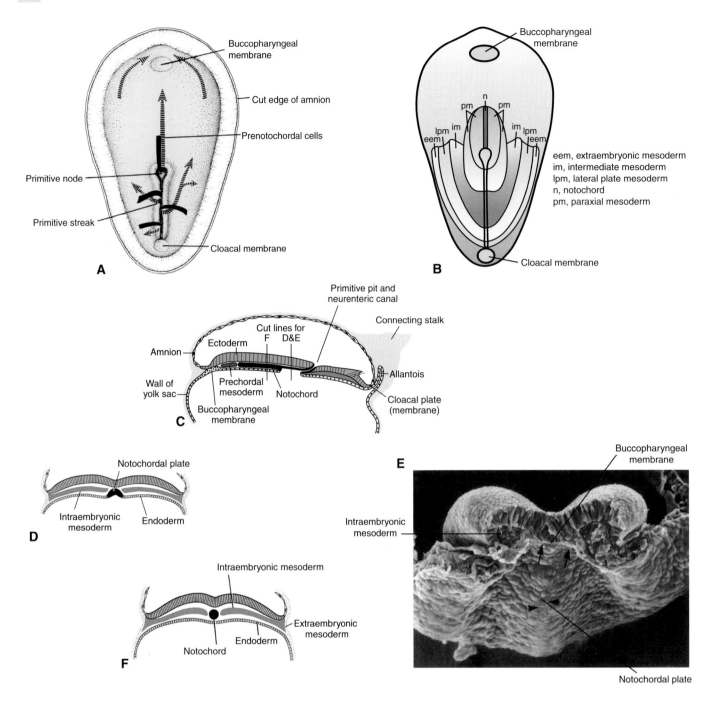

FIGURE 2.5. Epiblast cells migrate through the streak and node in specific patterns, such that their fate is determined by the region of the streak through which they pass (**A** and **B**). Thus, a "**fate map**" can be constructed showing that cells migrating through the most caudal aspect of the streak contribute to **extraembryonic mesoderm**, whereas those passing through in more cranial segments form **lateral plate**, **intermediate mesoderm**, and **paraxial mesoderm** (**B**). Some cells migrate through the most cranial aspect of the node; these form the **prechordal plate mesoderm** and **notochord** (**A** and **B**). Cells destined to form prechordal plate mesoderm migrate before notochordal cells and assume a position between the buccopharyngeal membrane and the cranial end of the notochord (**C**). Later, these cells are important for inducing forebrain development (Chapter 9; Fig. 9.10H). Notochordal cells follow those destined to form prechordal mesoderm and, at first, intercalate themselves in the endoderm layer to form the notochordal plate (**D** and **E**). Later, they detach to form the definitive notochord, a tight column of cells in close approximation to the floor of the neural tube, extending from the prechordal plate cranially to the tail bud caudally (**F**). The notochord establishes the midline and sends molecular signals essential for induction of the neural tube, somites, and other surrounding structures (Chapter 9; Fig. 9.10A–F). Only two parts of the original bilaminar disc do not become trilaminar—the **buccopharyngeal membrane** (plate) cranially and the **cloacal membrane** (plate) caudally (**B**). In these regions, epiblast and hypoblast remain tightly adherent to each other. Later, these membranes break down to form openings into the oral cavity and anus, respectively.

Dorsal Views of Gastrulating Embryos

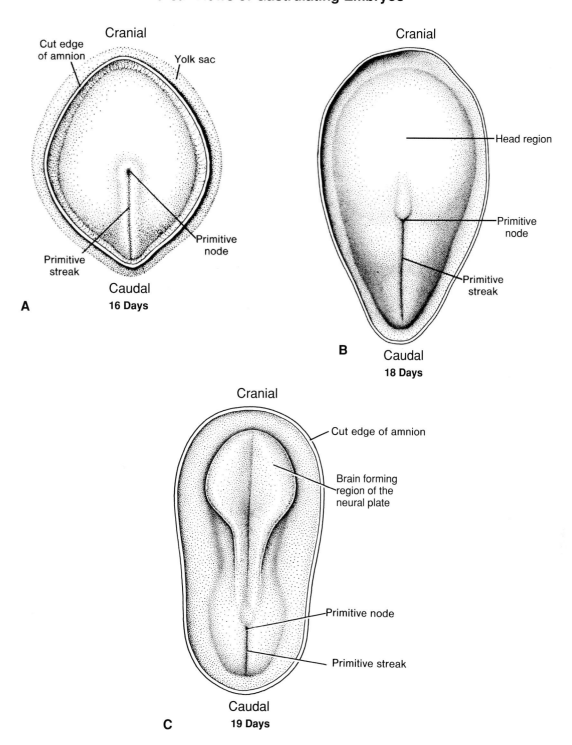

FIGURE 2.6.   The process of gastrulation continues for almost 2 weeks, beginning on day 16 (**A**) and ending just before closure of the caudal-most part of the neural tube on day 28. It proceeds in a cranial to caudal sequence, with head mesoderm forming first (**B** and **C**). In fact, induction of the brain and cranial portion of the spinal cord is initiated at the same time that gastrulation continues in more caudal segments (**C**). Thus, the formation of embryonic structures typically is more advanced in cranial regions than in caudal regions of the embryo.

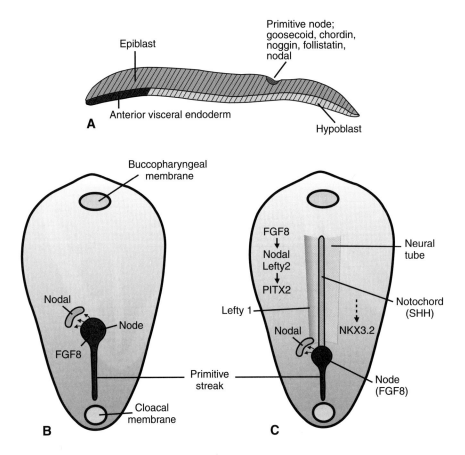

FIGURE 2.7. The third week also is characterized by establishment of the craniocaudal, dorsoventral, and right–left axes in the embryo. Molecular signals from genes regulating head development are expressed first in the **anterior visceral endoderm** (part of the hypoblast) and establish the cranial end of the embryo (**A**; this figure illustrates a midline section through the length of the embryonic disc). These genes include the transcription factors *OTX2, LIM1,* and *HESX1.* Once the head end is established, the primitive streak forms caudally. The streak is established and maintained by expression of *nodal,* a member of the *transforming growth factor β (TGFβ)* gene family that soon appears in the primitive node-forming region. Once the craniocaudal axis is formed, dorsoventral polarity also is delineated. Another member of the *TGFβ* family, bone morphogenetic protein 4 (BMP4), is secreted throughout the embryonic disc (shown as the hatched area in **A**), and together with fibroblast growth factor (FGF), it ventralizes mesoderm into intermediate and lateral plate mesoderm. Inhibition of BMP4 dorsalizes mesoderm to form notochord, somites, and somitomeres (paraxial mesoderm). Genes that cause this inhibition include *goosecoid, noggin,* and *follistatin,* and expression of these genes occurs in the primitive node. Because it regulates these and other events, the node is called the "**organizer.**" Establishment of the left–right axis also involves the node and primitive streak (**B** and **C**). FGF8, secreted by the node, causes expression of *nodal* in mesoderm on the left side of the embryo. In turn, *nodal* initiates a cascade of gene expression on the left, including *lefty2* and the transcription factor *PITX2.* Meanwhile, expression of *lefty1* on the left side of the neural plate, together with *sonic hedgehog* expression in the notochord, blocks the expression of this cascade on the right. By some still undetermined mechanism, this expression pattern regulates left-sidedness. Genes regulating right-sidedness are mostly unknown, but the transcription factor *NKX3.2* plays a role. Individuals sometimes have a complete reversal of sidedness, a condition called **situs inversus**. In this situation, the heart is on the right, the liver on the left, and so on. In other cases, only a partial reversal of organ placement occurs, such that a person is predominantly left- or right-sided. The spleen reflects the differences, with those who are predominantly right-sided having asplenia (absent spleen) or hypoplastic (small) spleen and those who are predominantly left-sided having polysplenia. These conditions are known as **laterality sequences**. Patients with complete situs inversus usually do not have other abnormalities, whereas those with laterality sequences often have other birth defects, especially involving the heart.

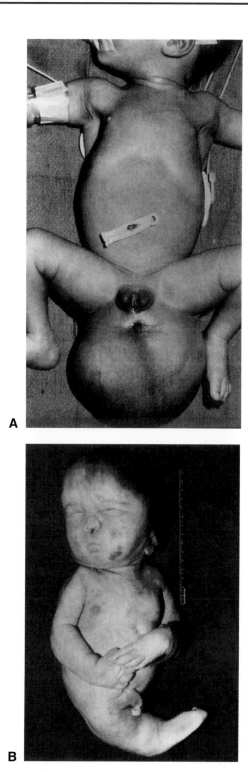

FIGURE 2.8. Other abnormalities also occur during gastrulation. A **sacrococcygeal teratoma** (A) is a tumor located in the sacrococcygeal region that apparently arises from continued proliferation and migration of epiblast cells through the primitive streak beyond the time when the caudal-most regions of the embryo have formed. Because these cells have the potential to form all three germ layers, derivatives of all of these layers are present in the tumors, including hair, skin, bone, liver, and so on. In contrast, if epiblast cells stop their migration too soon, insufficient mesoderm is produced and caudal structures cannot develop. This situation leads to **caudal dysgenesis**, in which, in its most severe expression, the lower limbs are fused, causing **sirenomelia** (B). Infants with this condition usually die due to renal agenesis, because there is insufficient intermediate mesoderm, and the kidneys fail to form. Caudal dysgenesis is more common in infants from insulin-dependent diabetic mothers and has been produced experimentally in mice through misexpression of the growth factor WNT and related genes.

CHAPTER 3

Neurulation and Establishment of Body Form

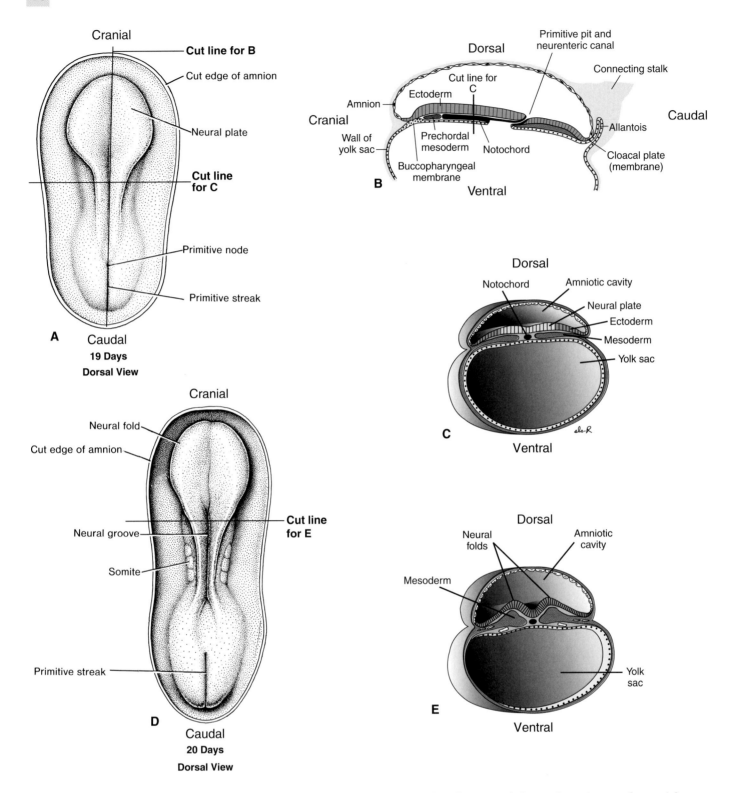

FIGURE 3.1. During the third and fourth weeks, the neural and gut tubes form, and the embryo is transformed from a trilaminar disc into the more recognizable embryo in the fetal position. The **neural tube** forms dorsally, as the ectoderm layer rolls up into a tube, while the gut tube forms ventrally, as the body folds downward (see Fig. 3.5). In this manner, "a tube on top of a tube" is created: the neural tube above, which differentiates into the brain and spinal cord, and the gut tube below, from the pharynx to the hindgut. Mesoderm then holds the two tubes together. The neural tube begins to develop at the middle of the third week, when ectoderm overlying prechordal mesoderm and the notochord is **induced** by these structures to form the **neural plate** (**A** and **B**). In essence, this plate represents a **placode**—a thickening of ectoderm caused by cells becoming tall and columnar as opposed to cuboidal (**C**). As with all development, induction occurs in the cranial region first, followed by more caudal segments. Once a neural plate is induced, the process of creating a neural tube, called **neurulation**, begins on day 20 of development. Cells in the neural plate elongate, and the lateral edges begin to elevate and curl toward the midline. This movement creates a groove in the midline, the **neural groove**, which is flanked by the elevating sides of the original neural plate that are now called the **neural folds** (**D** and **E**). These folds are larger in the cranial region, but become narrower in the hindbrain and spinal cord.

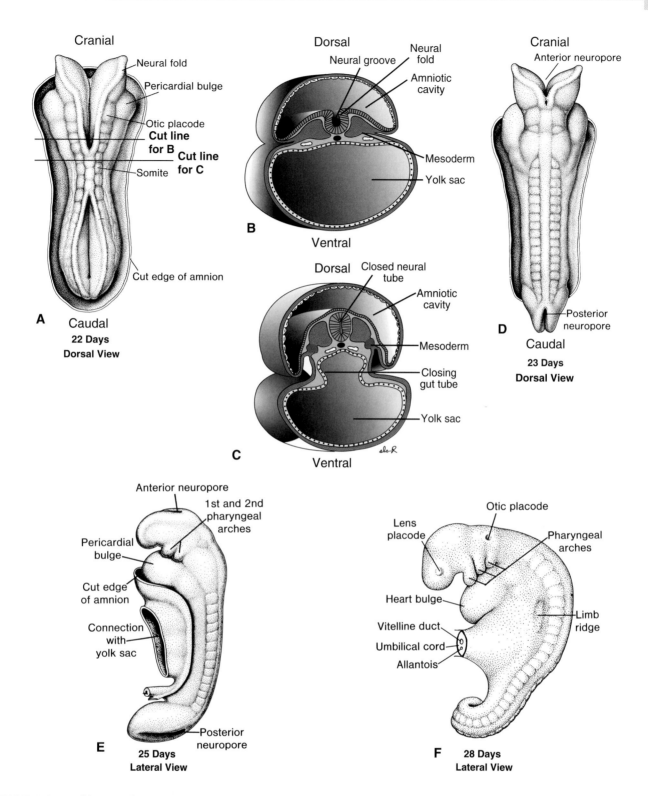

FIGURE 3.2. Folding (rolling up) of the neural plate continues until contact between opposing neural folds is achieved and a closed neural tube is formed. Contact between the folds is initiated in the cervical region, and zippering then occurs cranially and caudally until the tube is closed (**A–D**). Before the zippering process is complete, but after the folds have made initial contact, the prospective neural tube has openings cranially and caudally, the **anterior** and **posterior neuropores**, respectively (**D** and **E**). Closure of the anterior neuropore occurs on day 25; closure of the posterior neuropore occurs on day 28, again reflecting the cranial to caudal sequence of development (**E** and **F**).

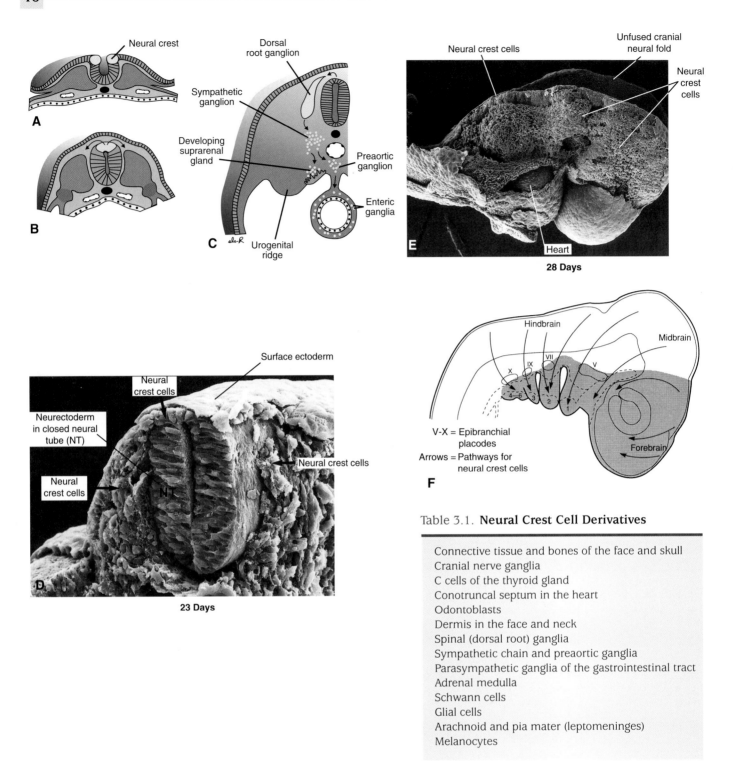

Table 3.1. Neural Crest Cell Derivatives

Connective tissue and bones of the face and skull
Cranial nerve ganglia
C cells of the thyroid gland
Conotruncal septum in the heart
Odontoblasts
Dermis in the face and neck
Spinal (dorsal root) ganglia
Sympathetic chain and preaortic ganglia
Parasympathetic ganglia of the gastrointestinal tract
Adrenal medulla
Schwann cells
Glial cells
Arachnoid and pia mater (leptomeninges)
Melanocytes

FIGURE 3.3.   As the neural folds elevate toward fusion, a new population of cells differentiates at the crest of the folds (**A**). These **neural crest cells** develop in the neurectoderm and migrate as fibroblast-like cells from the neural folds to form many structures (**B–D**; Table 3.1). In the spinal cord region, crest cells migrate after fusion of the folds (**C** and **D**), but in the cranial area they leave before fold closure (**E** and **F**). As they leave the neural folds, crest cells lose their ectodermal (epithelial) characteristics and become fibroblast-like, forming a loose connective tissue called **mesenchyme**. Later, after they reach their final destinations, they differentiate into a wide variety of cell types, some of which may be epithelial in nature (Table 3.1). Thus, crest cells begin as ectoderm (epithelial), transform to fibroblasts (mesenchyme), and then some become epithelial again (e.g., ganglia), while others remain mesenchymal, giving rise to derivatives characteristic of this tissue (connective tissue and bones of the face). Such transformations are not unique to neural crest cells. For example, some mesoderm cells begin with fibroblast characteristics (mesenchyme), then become epithelial (e.g., somites), and, finally, transform back to mesenchyme as they form definitive structures. (Note that the term mesenchyme refers to loose connective tissue regardless of origin, whereas mesoderm refers to one of the primary germ layers.)

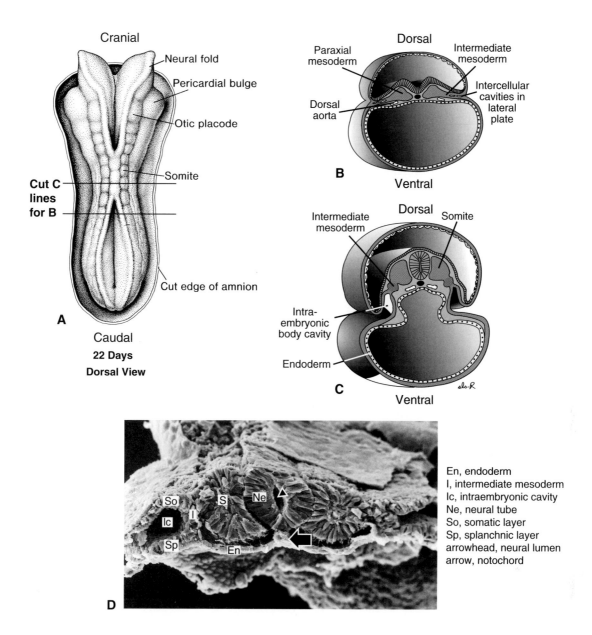

FIGURE 3.4. As the neural tube rolls up dorsally, the embryo also folds ventrally to form the gut tube and body cavities (see Fig. 3.5). Forces responsible for this folding are not clear, but proliferation of mesoderm and its rearrangement into paraxial, intermediate, and lateral plate components are involved. **Paraxial mesoderm** is located along the sides of the neural tube, i.e., along the axis of the embryo. It becomes organized into a series of segmentally arranged blocks called **somites** from the occipital region caudalward (**A–D**). In the head region, paraxial mesoderm forms more loosely organized collections of cells called **somitomeres**. Later these structures differentiate into part of the skull, vertebrae, muscles, and dermis of the skin (Fig. 4.1). **Intermediate mesoderm** lies between paraxial and lateral plate mesoderm (**C** and **D**). It is segmented cranially, but loses this segmentation in the lumbosacral regions where it will contribute to the urogenital system (Chapter 7). **Lateral plate mesoderm** lies at the lateral edges of the embryonic disc and will split into two layers: an outer **somatic (parietal)** and an inner **splanchnic (visceral) layer** (**B–D**). The visceral (organs) layer overlies the gut tube and all of its derivatives; the parietal (wall) layer lines the inside of the body wall. The space between the two layers forms what is initially called the **intraembryonic cavity**, but will eventually become the **definitive body cavities** (thorax, abdomen, and pelvis; **C** and Fig. 3.6). The two layers become very thin to form the **serous membranes** that secrete a fluid that moistens and lubricates the organs and body wall.

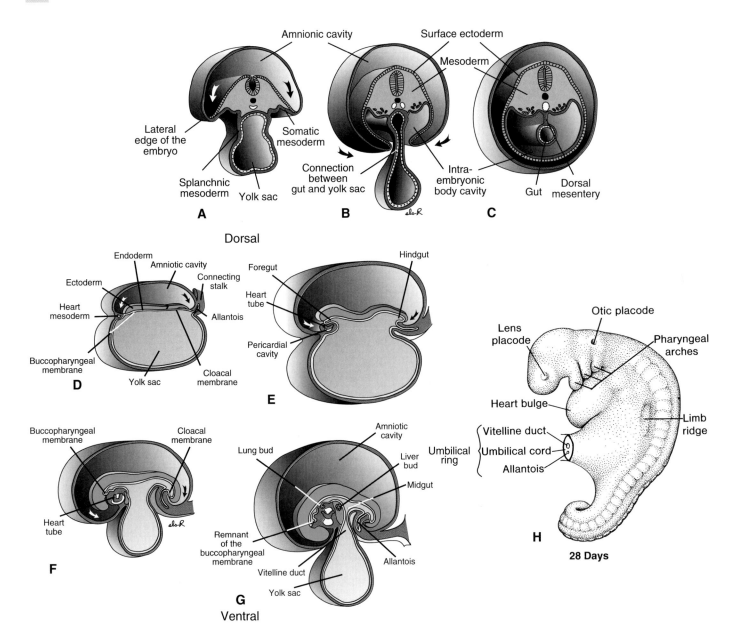

FIGURE 3.5. As proliferation and differentiation of the mesoderm continue, ventral folding occurs along the sides of the embryonic axis; hence, the sides moving downward are called **lateral folds** (**A**, *arrows*). This folding accomplishes three things: (1) it causes the endoderm layer to roll into a tube, the **gut tube** (**A–C**); (2) it pulls the amnion, which is attached to the lateral edges of the embryonic disc, ventrally so that it surrounds the embryo (**A–G**); and (3) together with the head and tail folds (**D–F**, *arrows*), it closes the ventral body wall around the **umbilical ring**, causing the embryo to assume a curved "fetal position" (**D–H**). These **head** and **tail folds** are similar to the lateral folds except that they occur at the cranial and caudal ends of the embryo (**D–F**, *arrows*). They are created by growth of the brain and lengthening of the embryonic axis. In essence, the four folds (head, tail, and two lateral) act like a purse string to draw the ventral body wall into a narrow region around the yolk sac and connecting stalk called the umbilical ring (**H**). As this region narrows, the opening of the gut tube into the yolk sac becomes smaller, and the connection forms the **vitelline (yolk sac) duct** (**G** and **H**). This connection persists until later in development (12 weeks) when the yolk sac degenerates. Blood vessels form in the connecting stalk, and this structure becomes the umbilical cord.

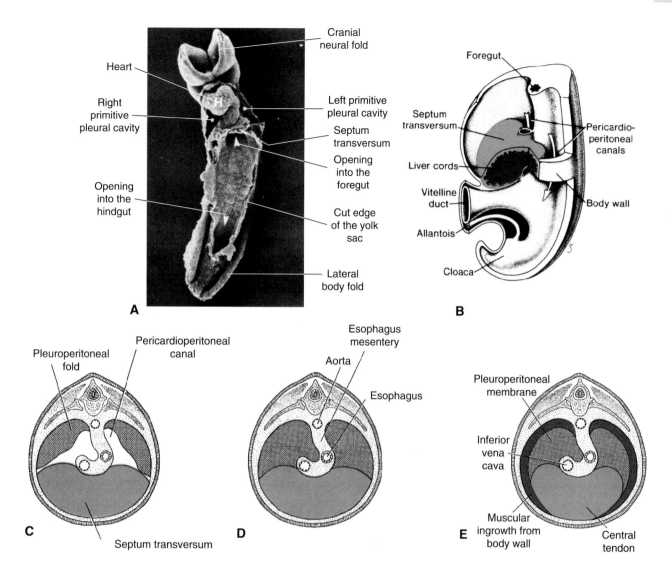

FIGURE 3.6. Once folding and neural tube closure have occurred on day 28, the embryo can be viewed as consisting of a tube on top of a tube. The neural tube, derived from ectoderm, lies dorsal to the gut tube, derived from endoderm. Mesoderm, the middle germ layer, surrounds each tube and holds them together (Fig. 3.5C). The primitive intraembryonic body cavity extends from thorax to pelvis and is not yet subdivided. Division of the intraembryonic cavity into thorax and abdomen is accomplished partially by mesoderm associated with the heart. The heart is derived from splanchnic (visceral) mesoderm at the cranial-most aspect of the embryonic disc (Fig. 3.5D). As the brain develops and lengthens, it overgrows this cardiac region, creating the head fold. In turn, growth of the head fold causes the heart to assume a more ventral and caudal position, moving it into a region that ultimately becomes the thorax (Fig. 3.5E–G). As these events occur, mesoderm caudal to the heart proliferates to form a thickened block of tissue called the **septum transversum** (A and B; see also Fig. 3.5G). This structure lies between the prospective thorax and abdomen and extends from the ventral body wall to the gut tube, but does not reach the posterior body wall (A and B). Here two canals, the **pericardioperitoneal canals**, on either side of the gut tube, remain to connect the primitive thoracic and peritoneal cavities (A). During the next several days, mesoderm of the septum transversum thins to form the **central tendon** of the **diaphragm** (C–E). Meanwhile, two membranes, the **pleuroperitoneal membranes**, grow from the posterior body wall to fuse with the septum transversum, thereby closing the pericardioperitoneal canals and separating the thoracic and peritoneal cavities (C and D). Later, muscle tissue, migrating from the body wall, covers the pleuroperitoneal membranes to form the muscular portion of the diaphragm (E).

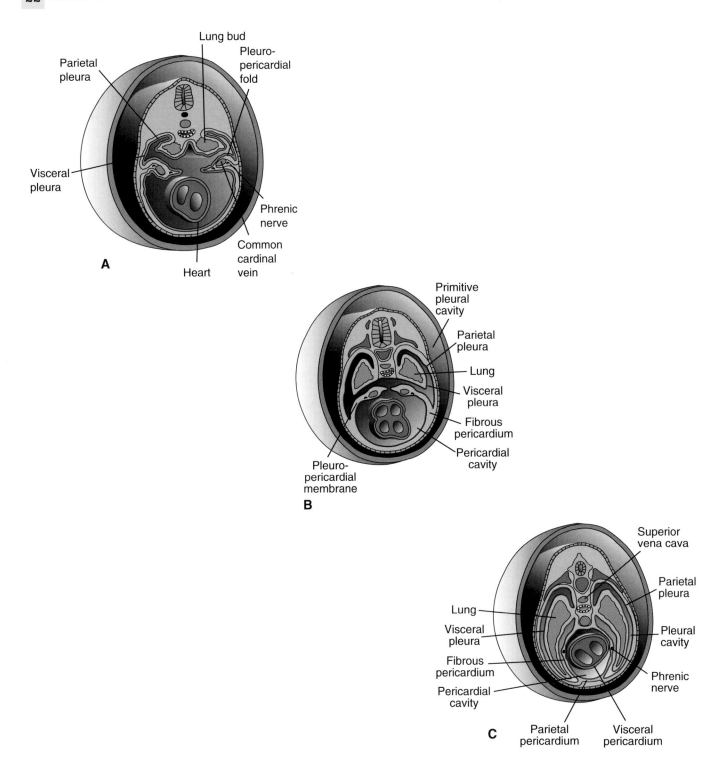

FIGURE 3.7.   The thoracic cavity separates into cardiac and pleural cavities when paired **pleuropericardial membranes** grow out from the lateral body wall and fuse in the midline (**A–C**). Because these membranes grow from the body wall, they carry structures that once were in the wall with them. In this case, the **phrenic nerves** to the diaphragm and the **common cardinal veins** are brought toward the midline (**B** and **C**) as these membranes surround the heart (**C**). Eventually, the pleuropericardial membranes become fibrous and form the **fibrous pericardium**, trapping the phrenic nerve in this structure (**C**).

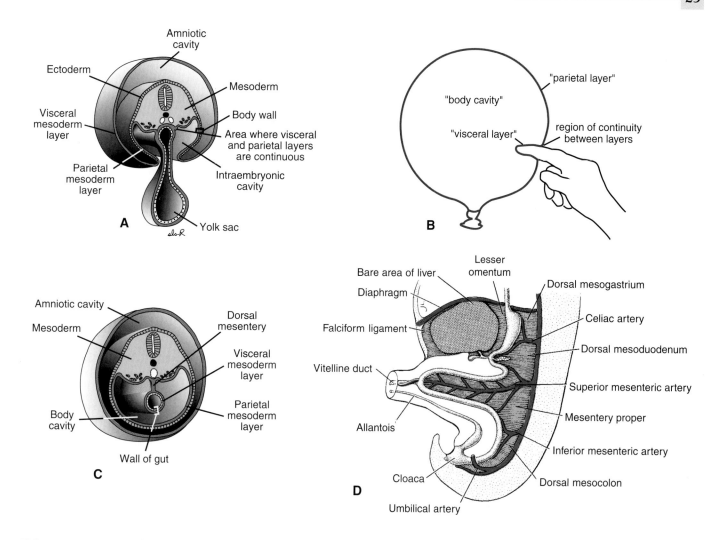

FIGURE 3.8. **Lateral plate mesoderm** lines the body cavity, and the portion covering organs forms a **visceral layer**, while the layer against the body wall forms a **parietal layer** (**A**). Organs are covered by the visceral layer as they grow into the body cavity (see lung bud; Fig. 3.7A) and this layer then takes the name of the organ involved. For example, that surrounding the lungs forms the visceral pleura; that around the heart, the visceral pericardium, and so on (Fig. 3.7C). The parietal layer on the body wall surrounding these organs then becomes the parietal pleura, parietal pericardium, and other parietal structures (Fig. 3.7C.) The heart has an additional layer, the fibrous pericardium, derived from the pleuropericardial membranes that separate the pleural and cardiac cavities (Fig. 3.7A–C). Both the visceral and parietal layers are continuous where the visceral layer reflects from the organ onto the body wall (**A;** see also Fig. 3.7A). The situation is analogous to having someone push a finger into an inflated balloon (Fig. 3.7B). The finger would be covered by a "visceral layer," while the outside layer (wall) of the balloon would form the "parietal layer." The space between the balloon and the finger would represent the primitive body cavity, and the two layers would be continuous at the base ("root") of the finger (**B**). In some regions of the gut tube, this continuation between visceral and parietal layers becomes thin and extended into a double-layered membrane, called a **mesentery**, that suspends portions of the gut from the **dorsal body wall** (**C** and **D**). Each mesentery is named according to the organ or portion of the gut to which it is attached, e.g., the dorsal mesogastrium (stomach), dorsal mesoduodenum, and dorsal mesocolon (**D**). In addition to forming attachments and support for organs, mesenteries provide a pathway for lymphatics, blood vessels, and nerves that pass from the body wall between the two layers to reach the organs they supply (**D**). A **ventral mesentery** attaching the gut tube to the ventral body wall also forms (from thinning of the septum transversum), but only in the segment of the gut extending from the stomach to the upper end of the duodenum (**D**). Later, as the liver grows into the septum transversum, this ventral mesentery is divided into the lesser omentum, extending from the liver to the stomach and upper duodenum, and the falciform ligament, extending from the liver to the ventral body wall (**D;** Fig. 6.3).

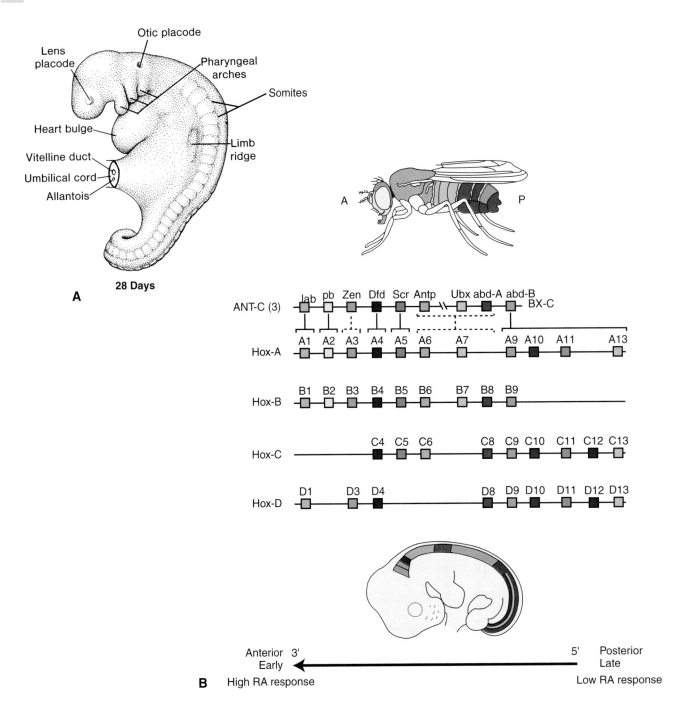

FIGURE 3.9. After neural tube closure and body folding are complete, most of the embryo is segmented. Segmentation is especially recognizable by the organization of somites along the neural tube (**A**), but other examples include the pharyngeal arches (**A**; see also Fig. 8.1) and the hindbrain (see Fig. 9.10G). This patterning is sequentially arranged along the cranial to caudal axis. Interestingly, regulation of this patterning involves the same genes used to regulate cranial to caudal development in *Drosophila* (fruit flies). These **homeobox (HOX) genes** code for a family of **transcription factors** that share a common DNA-binding motif called the **homeodomain**. In *Drosophila*, the *hox* genes belong to the *Antennapedia* (*ANT-C*) and *Bithorax* (*BX-C*) classes and are arranged in a linear sequence along the 3′ to 5′ axis of a single chromosome (**B**). During evolution, these genes have been duplicated such that humans have four groups of *HOX* genes located on four different chromosomes (**B**; homology between *Drosophila* genes and clusters of human genes are indicated by color. Genes with the same number, but positioned on different chromosomes, form a **paralogous** group). Expression of the genes is in a cranial to caudal direction from the 3′ (expressed early) to 5′ (expressed later) end, as indicated in the fly and mouse diagrams. By using overlapping patterns of expression among the four groups of genes, patterning of vertebrae from somites (e.g., a cervical versus a thoracic vertebra) as well as that of other structures is specified. The genes themselves are responsive to **retinoic acid (RA)**, and this compound assists in regulating their expression, with genes at the 3′ end being more responsive than those toward the 5′ end (Fig. 3.9B). The fact that retinoic acid is involved in regulating these important genes is one reason why this compound and its derivatives, called retinoids, are so effective in causing birth defects (See Table 11.4).

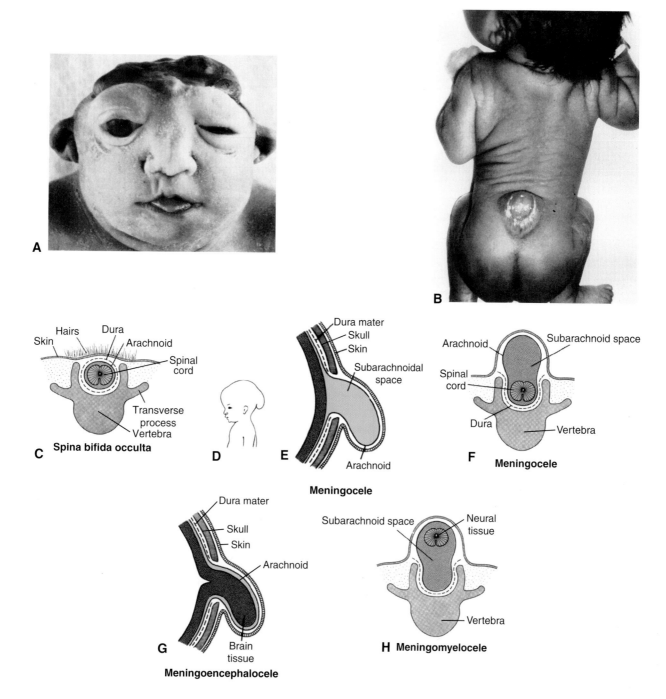

FIGURE 3.10. During neural tube closure and body folding, abnormalities may arise that result in birth defects. In some cases, the neural tube or bony structures surrounding it do not close properly, causing a spectrum of malformations called **neural tube defects**. In severe instances, opposing neural folds fail to fuse and remain divergent. This abnormality can occur anywhere along the tube, for varying distances. If the defect occurs cranially, it is called **anencephaly** (absent brain) because the two unfused folds degenerate, leaving little or no brain tissue and resulting in death of the child (**A**). If the abnormality occurs along the spinal cord, it is called **spina bifida cystica**. The most common site for this defect is in the lumbosacral area (**B**). Some degree of paralysis occurs depending on the level of the lesion, but these children survive. In 10% of individuals, the neural tube closes normally, but the vertebrae remain bifid and do not form a neural arch around the spinal cord (**C**). Again, the most common site for this abnormality is in the lumbosacral area, where it may be covered by skin having a patch of dark hair. This defect, called **spina bifida occulta**, causes no functional deficits. Other defects include meningoceles (**D–F**), meningoencephaloceles (**E** and **G**), and meningomyeloceles (**H**). In all these cases there is a bony defect in either the skull or vertebrae through which meninges covering the brain or spinal cord protrude. If only meninges are involved, the defect is called a meningocele; if the defect includes brain tissue, it is called an encephalocele; and if it includes spinal cord tissue, it is called a myelomeningocele. Neural tube defects occur in approximately 1 per 1000 births, although rates may be much higher in different areas. It is essential to remember that up to 70% of these defects can be prevented if a woman takes 400 μg of **folic acid** a day (usually as a multivitamin supplement) beginning 2 to 3 months prior to conception and then throughout gestation.

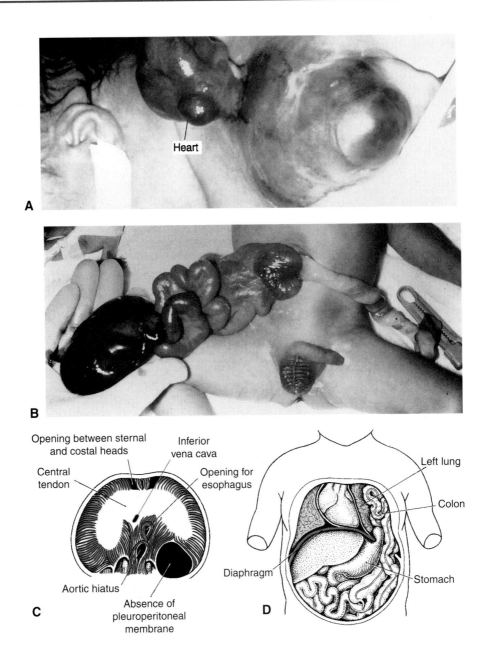

FIGURE 3.11. Birth defects also arise because of abnormalities in ventral body wall closure, resulting in **ventral body wall defects**. Failure of the head folds and lateral body folds to close in the midline causes cleft sternum. If the defect is severe, the heart lies outside the thoracic cavity, a condition called ectopia cordis (**A**). The defect also may extend into the abdomen, creating a spectrum of abnormalities that includes cleft sternum, ectopia cordis, heart defects, anterior diaphragmatic hernias, and omphalocele (herniated bowel loops protruding through the umbilicus; see Fig. 6.7G and H). **Gastroschisis** is another ventral body wall defect in which loops of bowel herniate through the abdominal wall lateral to the umbilicus, usually on the right side (**B**). It is not clear whether this defect is due to a folding problem or to a weakening in this region. Problems with partitioning the body cavity also may arise in the form of **diaphragmatic hernias**. Most hernias (85%–90%) occur on the left posterior side because of failure of the pleuroperitoneal membrane to grow and close the left pericardioperitoneal canal (**C**). Abdominal viscera may herniate into the thorax and, if the defect is extensive, compress the lungs and displace the heart, leading to fetal death (**D**). Less commonly, other smaller defects in the diaphragm occur anteriorly (parasternal hernias) or around the esophagus (esophageal hernia; **C**).

CHAPTER 4

Musculoskeletal System

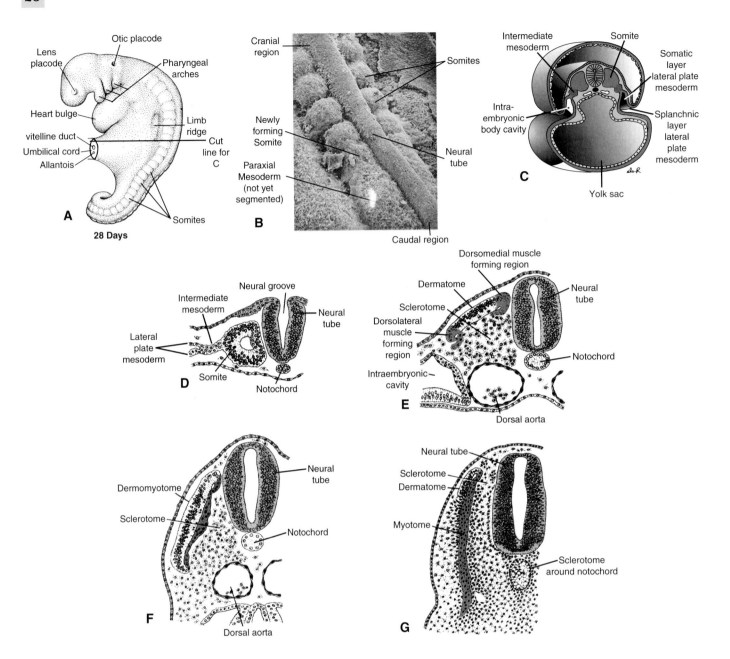

FIGURE 4.1. The **skeletal system** develops from **paraxial and lateral plate (somatic layer) mesoderm** and from **neural crest cells**. The **muscular system** consists of **skeletal, smooth, and cardiac** types. **Skeletal muscle** is derived from paraxial mesoderm; **smooth muscle** differentiates from the splanchnic layer of lateral plate mesoderm surrounding the gut and its derivatives; and **cardiac muscle** develops from the splanchnic layer of lateral plate mesoderm surrounding the heart tube. In addition, smooth muscle for the pupil, mammary glands, and sweat glands differentiates from ectoderm. Clearly, paraxial mesoderm plays a key role in forming both the skeletal and muscular systems. This mesoderm-derived tissue, lying along the axis of the embryo, becomes organized into segmentally arranged clusters that are called **somitomeres** in the head and **somites** (**A–C**) from the occipital region to the coccyx. The process of segmentation begins with paraxial mesoderm forming loose collections of mesenchymal cells. Somitomeres retain this pattern, but somites become further organized into discrete epithelial segments (**D**) on either side of the neural tube (spinal column), with more cranially placed units forming before more caudal units (**B**). At this stage (4 weeks), somites appear as pairs of donut-shaped structures (**D**). As development proceeds, the ventromedial portion of each somite becomes mesenchymal again and forms the **sclerotome** (**E**). These are bone-forming cells. The dorsolateral and dorsomedial portions of the somite form muscle cells. Those from the dorsolateral region migrate to form limb and body wall muscles (**hypomeric musculature; E**), whereas dorsomedial cells migrate beneath the remaining dorsal potion of the somite to form muscles of the back (**epimeric musculature; E–G**). The dorsal-most region of the somite forms the **dermatome** that migrates and differentiates into the **dermis** of the skin (**E–G**). Together, muscle cells from the dorsomedial part of the somite and the dermatome form the **dermomyotome** (**F**).

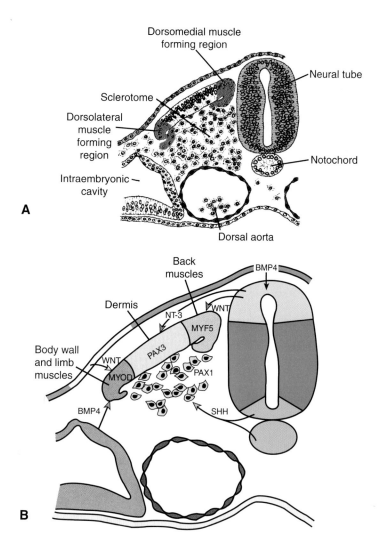

FIGURE 4.2. Molecular regulation of somite differentiation relies on a complex series of genetic signals from surrounding tissues. Sonic hedgehog (SHH), a secreted signal molecule expressed in the floor plate of the neural tube and the notochord, initiates *PAX1* expression in presumptive sclerotome cells, and this transcription factor regulates differentiation of these cells into bone (**A** and **B**). Expression of the growth factor bone morphogenetic protein 4 (BMP4), by overlying ectoderm, causes secretion of WNT growth factors from the dorsal region of the neural tube. In turn, these growth factors cause expression of the muscle-specific gene *MYF5* in the dorsomedial portion of the somite, and this gene regulates development of epimeric (back) muscles. *WNT* proteins expressed by overlying ectoderm, together with BMP4 expressed by lateral plate mesoderm, turn on *MYOD* expression in the dorsolateral part of the somite. *MYOD* is another muscle-specific gene that causes this region to differentiate into limb and body wall muscles (hypomeric musculature). Dermis development is controlled by the transcription factor *PAX3,* the expression of which is initiated by the growth factor neurotrophin 3 (NT3), secreted by the dorsal region of the neural tube.

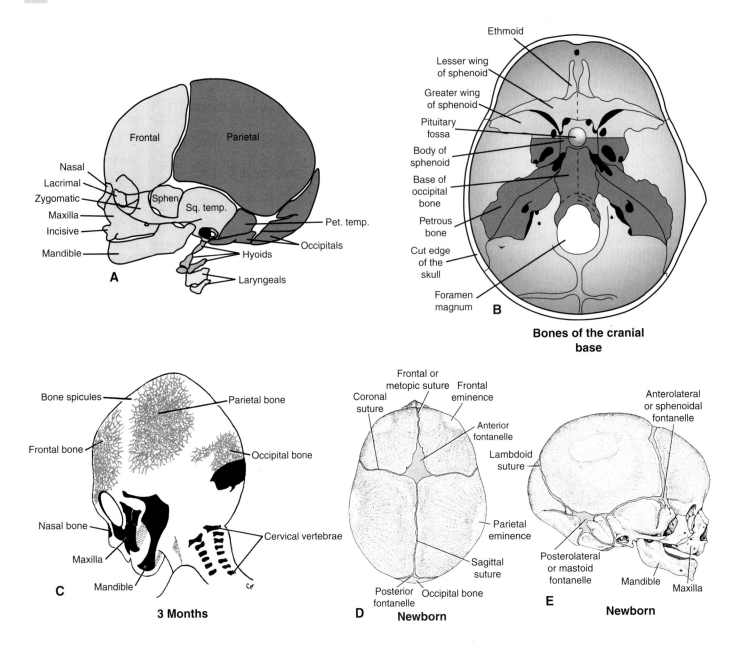

Bones of the cranial base

3 Months

Newborn

Newborn

FIGURE 4.3.   As mentioned previously, much of the skeletal system is derived from paraxial mesoderm that forms parts of the skull, the vertebrae, and ribs. The **skull** is divided into two parts: the **neurocranium**, which forms the protective covering for the brain, and the **viscerocranium**, which forms the skeleton of the face (**A**). The neurocranium also has two parts: the **membranous portion**, consisting of the flat bones around the brain (**A**); and the **cartilaginous portion**, or **chondrocranium**, which forms the base of the skull (**B**). Both parts of the neurocranium are derived from a combination of paraxial mesoderm (**A** and **B**; red) and neural crest cells (**A** and **B**; blue). In contrast, the entire viscerocranium is derived from neural crest (**A**). Cells contributing to the membranous portion of the neurocranium differentiate directly into bone by a process called **membranous ossification** (**C**), whereas the chondrocranium is formed by **endochondral ossification** whereby cells first establish a cartilaginous model for each bone, followed by ossification (**C**; see also page 33) for details on endochondral bone formation). As the flat bones form, they remain separated by narrow seams of connective tissue called **sutures** (**D** and **E**). In some areas, where more than two bones meet, sutures form wider regions called **fontanelles**. The largest of these is the **anterior fontanelle**, which forms the "soft spot" on the dorsal aspect of a baby's head. Sutures permit growth of the skull, to accommodate both pre- and postnatal growth of the brain, and overlap (moulding) of the bones as the baby passes through the birth canal. Some sutures remain unfused into adulthood, even though brain growth ceases within several years after birth. The degree of suture closure is used by forensic pathologists to help determine the age of skeletal remains.

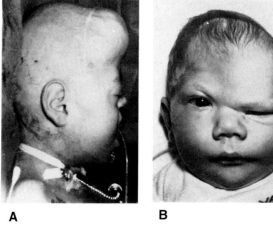

A   **B**

Table 4.1. **Genes Associated with Skeletal Defects**

Gene	Chromosome	Abnormality	Phenotype
FGFR1	8p12	Pfeiffer syndrome	Craniosynostosis, broad great toes and thumbs, cloverleaf skull, underdeveloped face
FGFR2	10q26	Pfeiffer syndrome	Same
		Apert syndrome	Craniosynostosis, underdeveloped face, symmetric syndactyly of hands and feet
		Jackson-Weiss syndrome	Craniosynostosis, underdeveloped face, no foot or hand defects
		Crouzon syndrome	Craniosynostosis, underdeveloped face, no foot or hand defects
FGFR3	4p16	Achondroplasia	Short-limb dwarfism, underdeveloped face
		Thanatophoric dysplasia (type I)	Curved short femurs, with or without cloverleaf skull
		Thanatophoric dysplasia (type II)	Milder form of achondroplasia with normal craniofacial features

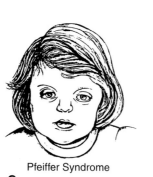

Pfeiffer Syndrome

C

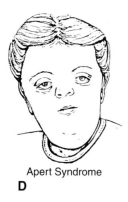

Apert Syndrome

D

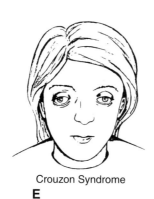

Crouzon Syndrome

E

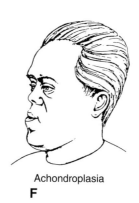

Achondroplasia

F

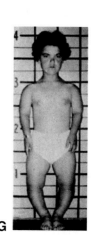

G

FIGURE 4.4.   Sometimes sutures fuse too early in development, resulting in **craniosynostosis** and abnormally shaped skulls. Final skull morphology depends on which suture or sutures are affected. For example, early closure of the sagittal suture results in scaphocephaly, a condition in which the skull is narrow with expanded frontal and occipital regions (**A**). Early closure of coronal and lambdoid sutures unilaterally results in plagiocephaly, in which one side of the skull is smaller than the other (**B**). If these conditions are not corrected by surgery, brain growth is affected severely. Recent advances in molecular genetics have shown that a family of growth factors called **fibroblast growth factors (FGFs)** and their **receptors (FGFRs)** are important for bone and cartilage development. Furthermore, mutations, particularly in the receptors, result in a number of syndromes involving craniosynostosis, facial development, and the limbs (**C–G**; Table 4.1). The types of defects that occur depend on which receptor is affected or where in the genetic sequence of a specific receptor a mutation occurs. This specificity explains why mutations in the same receptor can result in more than one phenotype. Other defects of the skull include anencephaly, in which the neural tube fails to close in the cranial region, resulting in partial or complete absence of the cranial vault (see page 25); and meningoceles and meningoencephaloceles, where smaller defects in the bony vault occur (see page 25).

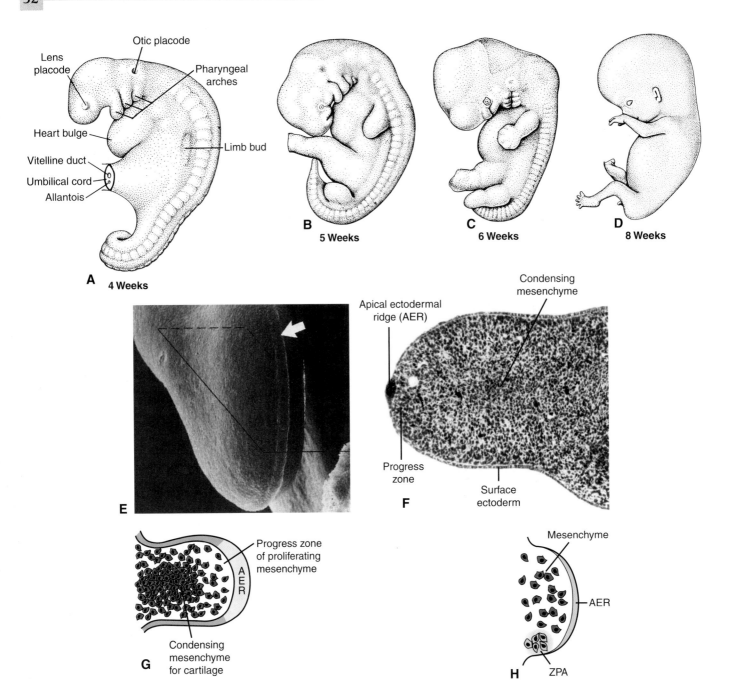

FIGURE 4.5. Limb development begins near the end of the fourth week, and limb morphology, complete with digits, is established by the eighth week (**A–D**). **Limb buds** appear as outgrowths from the flank at the end of the fourth week (**A**), with upper limbs appearing a day and a half before the lower limbs. Initially, the buds consist of a core of mesoderm, derived from the somatic layer of lateral plate mesoderm, covered by ectoderm. Soon, ectoderm at the limb tip proliferates and thickens to form the **apical ectodermal ridge (AER; E** and **F)**. This structure exerts an inductive influence on adjacent mesenchyme cells to maintain them as a rapidly proliferating, undifferentiated cell population called the **progress zone** (**F** and **G**). Maintenance of the progress zone causes the limb to elongate in a proximal to distal direction. As growth occurs, cells in the proximal part of the progress zone become positioned further from the AER and its influence. Consequently, these cells cease proliferation, condense into tighter groups, and begin to differentiate into the cartilaginous components of the limb. In this manner, the shoulder and pelvic girdles form first, followed by the long bones, and, finally, the digits. Thus, the AER regulates growth along the **proximal–distal limb axis**. Another regulating region of limb development is called the **zone of polarizing activity (ZPA)**, situated at the posterior border near the AER (**H**). The ZPA regulates limb patterning and growth in the **anterior (cranial)** to **posterior (caudal) direction** so that the thumb lies on the radial (anterior) side and the little finger lies on the ulnar (posterior) side.

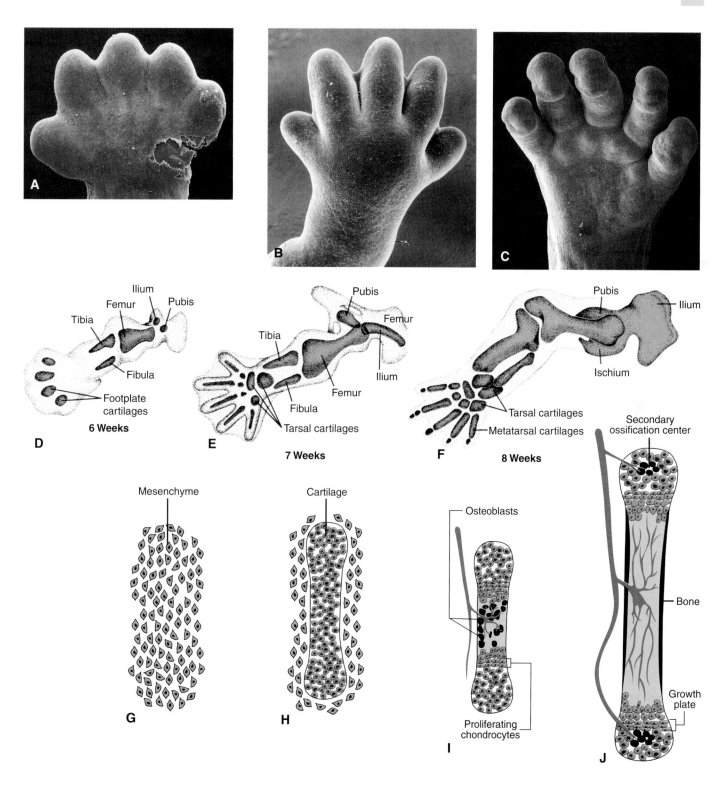

FIGURE 4.6. Digits form when **programmed cell death (apoptosis)** divides the AER into five segments to permit continued growth for each digit (**A**). Tissue remaining between digits also is subjected to programmed cell death to prevent webbing (**B** and **C**; ducks have no programmed cell death in their interdigital spaces). Bones in the limbs are derived from lateral plate (somatic layer) mesoderm and form by **endochondral ossification**. Thus, each bone is first patterned in cartilage by mesenchymal cells (**D–H**), followed by ossification, which is initiated in the shaft (**diaphysis; I**). Later, secondary ossification centers appear at the ends (**epiphyses**) of the bones (**J**). Bone growth is maintained by cartilage-forming regions, called **growth (epiphyseal) plates,** at the ends of the bones (**J**). These plates lie between the epiphyses and diaphyses and disappear (close) when growth is completed. Ossification begins in the eighth week, and primary ossification centers are present in all of the long bones by the twelfth week. Muscles for the limbs are derived from the dorsolateral portion of somites (paraxial mesoderm) in limb-forming regions. These cells migrate into the limbs, carrying their spinal nerves with them (see page 28), and differentiate into the complex pattern characteristic of limb musculature.

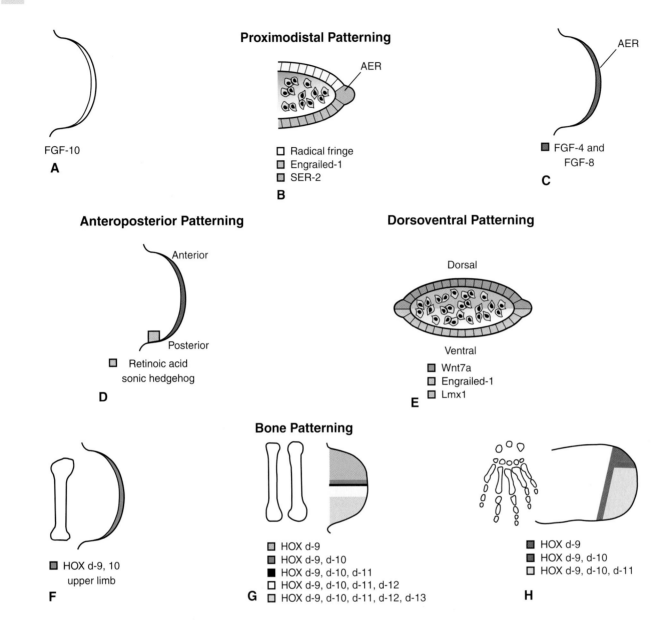

FIGURE 4.7. Molecular signals regulating limb development have been well characterized. Positioning along the cranial–caudal axis of the body is specified by *HOX* genes (see page 24). Outgrowth is initiated by fibroblast growth factor 10 (FGF10), secreted by the somatic layer of lateral plate mesoderm in limb-forming regions (**A**). The AER is induced by bone morphogenetic proteins (BMPs) secreted by ventral limb ectoderm. *Radical fringe,* expressed in dorsal limb ectoderm, restricts the AER to the distal tip by inducing expression of *SER2* at the border between dorsal and ventral limb ectoderm (**B**). The border is further defined by the expression boundaries of the transcription factor *Engrailed 1(EN1),* which blocks *Radical fringe* expression in ventral limb ectoderm (**B**). Once the AER is established, it secretes FGF4 and FGF8, which maintain the progress zone of mesoderm as a rapidly proliferating, undifferentiated cell population (**C**). Anterior–posterior patterning of the limb is regulated by the ZPA, a cluster of mesoderm cells located close to the AER in the posterior border of the limb (**D**). These cells produce retinoic acid, which, in turn, initiates expression of the secreted factor sonic hedgehog (SHH). SHH then acts as a morphogen to regulate patterning along this axis. Dorsoventral patterning is regulated by BMPs secreted by ventral limb ectoderm that induce expression of *EN1* (**E**). *EN1* represses *WNT7a* expression in ventral limb ectoderm, thereby restricting its presence to dorsal regions. Dorsally, *WNT7a* induces expression of *LMX1,* a homeodomain containing transcription factor that regulates dorsoventral development. Bone shapes are patterned by *HOX* genes expressed in complex, overlapping arrays (**F–H**), while the transcription factors *TBX4* and *5* regulate hindlimb and forelimb development, respectively.

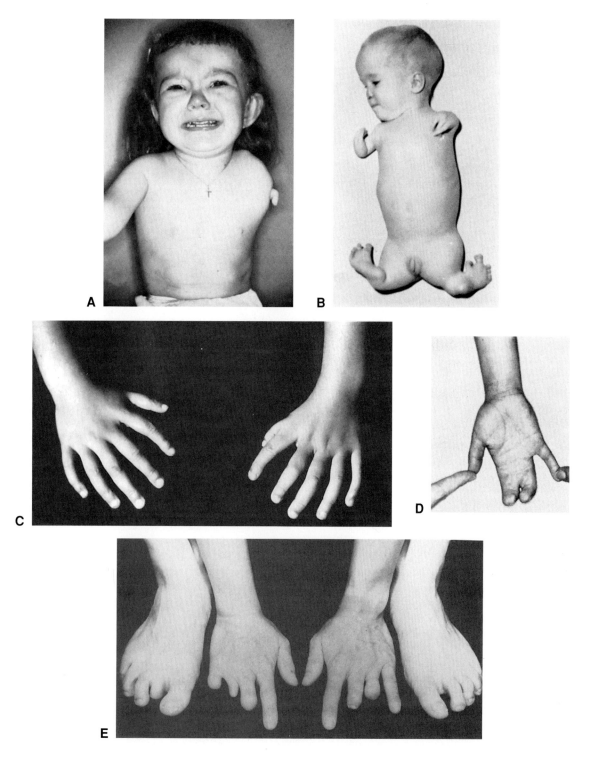

FIGURE 4.8. Many different types of birth defects involve the limbs. They may be caused by teratogens (e.g., chemicals, environmental agents) or by genetic mutations or combinations thereof. Most limb defects are induced during the early stages of development in the fourth or fifth week of gestation. One of the most potent limb teratogens is **thalidomide**, a drug once used as a sleeping pill and antinauseant and now employed in AIDS and cancer therapies. The drug causes a variety of limb defects, primarily involving the long bones. In some cases, exposure results in absent limbs (amelia; **A**), or shortened limbs (meromelia), or shortened limbs with feet or hands attached almost directly to the body, a form of meromelia called phocomelia (**B**). **Retinoids** are another class of teratogens that can produce all of these types of limb defects and others as well. Digital defects also occur, including polydactyly (extra digits; **C**), syndactyly (fused digits; **D**), ectrodactyly (absent digits), and brachydactyly (short digits). These defects have many causes. For example, the polydactyly in **C** shows a duplication of the middle digit and might be due to misexpression of SHH. Sometimes, amputations of the digits or limbs may occur due to amniotic bands that wrap around and constrict these structures as they are developing (**E**). **Amniotic bands** arise from pieces of amnion torn from the sac, either because of fetal movements or as scar tissue from in utero infections. In either case, the torn pieces form fibrous strands (bands) that become entangled in parts of the embryo, usually the limbs or face.

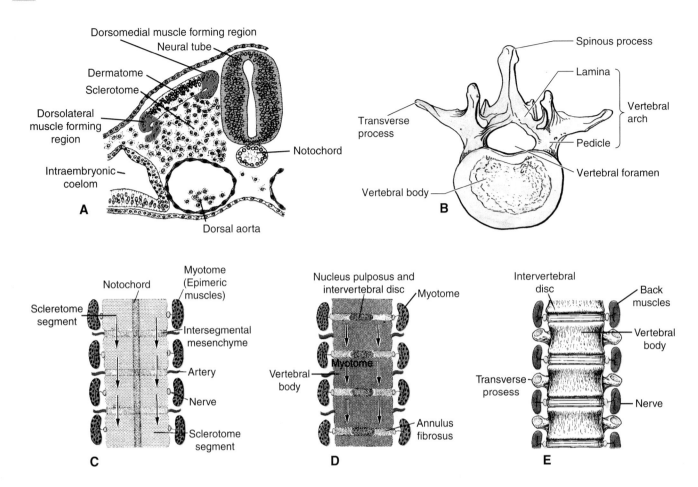

FIGURE 4.9. **Vertebrae** form from somites derived from paraxial mesoderm (**A**). Each vertebra consists of a **vertebral arch** and **foramen** (through which the spinal cord passes), a **body, transverse processes**, and, usually, a **spinous process** (**B**). All of these parts are derived from the **sclerotome** portion of the somites (**A**). During the fourth week, sclerotome cells migrate around the spinal cord and notochord to merge with sclerotome cells from the opposing somite on the other side of the neural tube (**A**). Cells in the caudal portion of each somite also grow caudally into the cranial half of each adjacent somite (**C**; *arrows*). Thus, the original segmental pattern of the somites, in which the sclerotome and myotome from each segment are aligned (**C**), becomes reorganized into a new segmental pattern, in which each vertebra is comprised of the caudal half of one somite and the cranial half of its neighbor (**D**; note positional change of arrows from **C** to **D**). In contrast, **myotomes** for **epimeric (back) musculature** retain their original position and, therefore, overlap adjacent vertebrae (**D**). This positioning allows the muscles to move the vertebral column at the vertebral joints. **Intervertebral discs** form between vertebrae (**D** and **E**) and consist of an outer ring, the **annulus fibrosis**, and a center filled with a gelatinous cushioning material, the **nucleus pulposus** (**D**). This central part of the disc is derived from proliferation of original notochord cells in the region of the discs (**A**). The remaining parts of the notochord degenerate. HOX gene expression regulates the shape of each vertebra. Ribs are also derivatives of paraxial mesoderm, since they grow out from the transverse processes of the thoracic vertebrae (**B**).

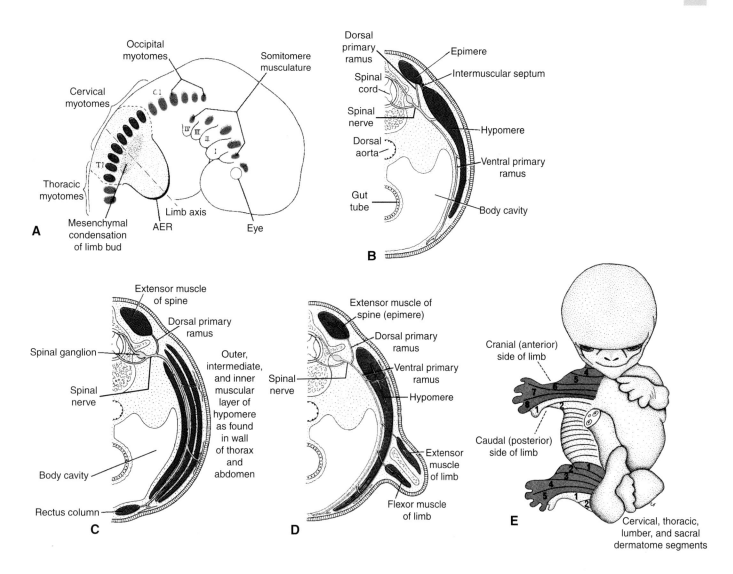

FIGURE 4.10. Somitomeres and somites form the musculature of the axial skeleton, body wall, and limbs (**A**; skeletal muscles). Somitomeres and the first few somites provide all of the head musculature (**A**; Table 4.2), except the pupillary muscles, which are derived from optic cup ectoderm (See page 120). At the end of the fifth week, each of the remaining somites has differentiated into two muscle-forming regions: a small dorsal portion, the **epimere** (**B**), formed from the dorsomedial cells of the somite that reorganized as myotomes (Fig. 4.9A); and a larger ventral part, the **hypomere** (**B**), formed by migration of dorsolateral cells of the original somites (Fig. 4.9A). Myoblasts of the epimere form muscles for the vertebral column (back muscles; **C**); while those of the hypomere give rise to muscles of the body wall (**C**; Table 4.3) and limbs (**D**). In addition, a ventral longitudinal muscle column forms at the tip of the hypomeres and differentiates into the rectus abdominis muscle (**C**) and the infrahyoid musculature in the cervical region. (In the thorax this column normally disappears, but may be represented by the sternalis muscle.) All of these skeletal muscles and the **dermatomes** overlying them are innervated by **spinal nerves**, such that derivatives of each somite are supplied by the nerve that originally served that somite. As muscles differentiate into epimeres (dorsally) and hypomeres (ventrally), each spinal nerve divides into a **dorsal primary ramus**, to serve epimere-derived muscles from that segment, and a **ventral primary ramus**, to innervate hypomere-derived muscles from that segment (**C** and **D**). Even when muscle cells migrate, they continue to be innervated by the spinal nerve from their segment of origin, such that the original segmental nature of this relationship is maintained. This phenomenon explains the segmental pattern of innervation of the muscles and dermatomes. In fact, dermatomes are defined as that region of the skin supplied by a single spinal nerve (**E**). However, this pattern becomes somewhat distorted in the limbs because as the limbs elongate, they rotate. The upper limb rotates 90 degrees laterally, positioning the thumb laterally; the lower limb rotates 90 degrees medially, placing the great toe medially. Muscle patterns along the vertebrae, body wall, and limbs are established by connective tissue cells derived from mesoderm from somites (vertebral muscles) and the somatic layer of lateral plate mesoderm (body wall and limbs). Muscle patterns in the head are regulated by neural crest–derived connective tissue. As mentioned previously, cardiac muscle is derived from splanchnic mesoderm surrounding the heart tube (see Fig. 5.1E and F), while smooth muscle in the wall of the gut and gut derivatives is derived from splanchnic mesoderm surrounding these structures (see Fig. 3.8C).

Table 4.2. **Origins of the Craniofacial Muscles**

Mesodermal Origin	Muscles	Innervation
Somitomeres 1,2	Superior, medial, ventral recti	Oculomotor (CN III)
Somitomere 3	Superior oblique	Trochlear (CN IV)
Somitomere 4	Jaw-closing	Trigeminal (CN V)
Somitomere 5	Lateral rectus	Abducens (CN VI)
Somitomere 6	Jaw-opening, and other second arch	Facial (CN VII)
Somitomere 7	Stylopharyngeus	Glossopharyngeal (CN IX)
Somites 1,2	Intrinsic laryngeals	Vagus (CN X)
Somites 2–5[a]	Tongue	Hypoglossal (CN XII)

[a]Somites 2–5 constitute the occipital group (somite 1 degenerates for the most part)
CN, cranial nerve

Table 4.3. **Muscles Derived from Hypomeres**

Hypomeres	Muscles
Cervical	Scalenes, geniohyoid, prevertebral
Thoracic	External, internal, and innermost intercostals and transversus thoracis
	External and internal obliques and tranversus abdominis
Lumbar	Quadratus lumborum
Sacral and coccygeal	Pelvic diaphragm and striated muscles of the anus

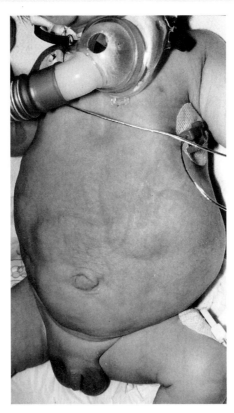

FIGURE 4.11.   Birth defects involving muscles are not common, although occasionally a muscle is missing. **Poland anomaly** is an example in which the pectoralis major muscle is absent unilaterally. This condition causes a marked deformity, especially for females. In another example, muscles of the abdominal wall are missing, resulting in **prune belly syndrome**. The syndrome is usually associated with urinary tract and bladder defects and may be secondary to abdominal distention caused by the urinary defects rather than agenesis of muscle tissue.

CHAPTER 5

Heart

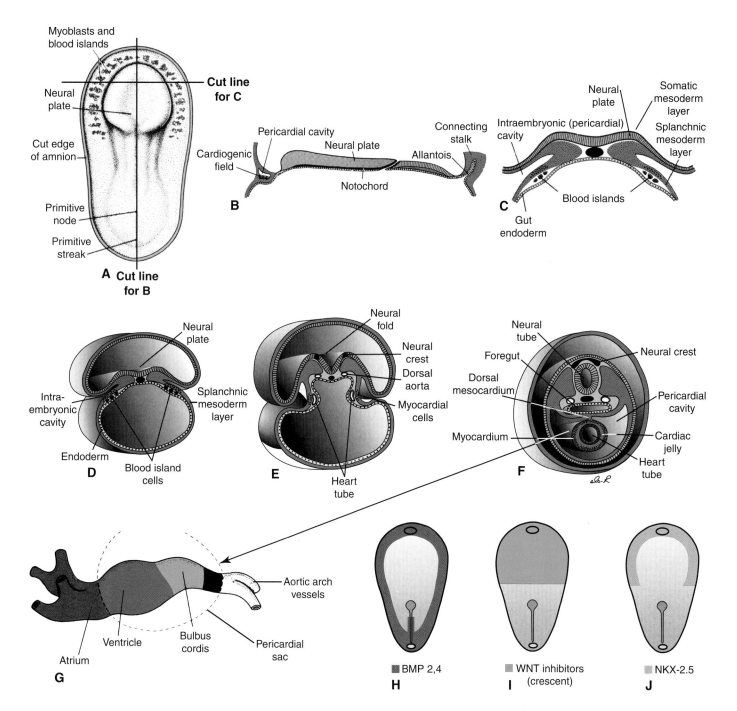

FIGURE 5.1. Heart development begins in the third week (18th day), when **blood islands** and **myoblasts** derived from **splanchnic mesoderm**, adjacent to gut endoderm, appear in a horseshoe-shaped region cranial to the neural plate (**A–C**). Soon, blood island cells coalesce to form a horseshoe-shaped endothelial tube that becomes surrounded by myocardial muscle cells. During the fourth week, caudal poles of the horseshoe are brought together in the midline by lateral folding of the embryonic disc, creating a single **heart tube** (**D–F**). During this process, the tube itself becomes segregated into regions of the **bulbus cordis, primitive ventricle (*left*)**, and **common atrium** (**G**). The bulbus cordis eventually gives rise to the **right ventricle, conus cordis**, and **truncus arteriosus**. Meanwhile, the cranial end of the tube sprouts blood vessels, called **aortic arch vessels** (**G**), that course around the pharynx (see page 52); while the original caudal poles of the horseshoe receive venous drainage flowing into the common atrium (**G**). By the end of the fourth week, the tube begins to beat in a rhythmic fashion from atrium to ventricle, and the first blood cells begin to flow. Also, at this time, a wave of cells grows down from the atrial region over the myocardium to invest the heart in a third layer called the **epicardium**. (This layer also is called the **visceral pericardium**.) Heart induction in the horseshoe-shaped region is initiated by a cascade of molecular signals. First, the growth factor bone morphogenetic protein (BMP) is upregulated in endoderm and splanchnic mesoderm, while expression of another growth factor, WNT, is inhibited (**H** and **I**). This combination results in expression of the homeobox-containing transcription factor, *NKX2.5*, the master gene regulating heart induction and the homologue of the *tinman* gene in *Drosophila* (**J**; so-called because in *The Wizard of Oz*, the tinman was looking for a heart).

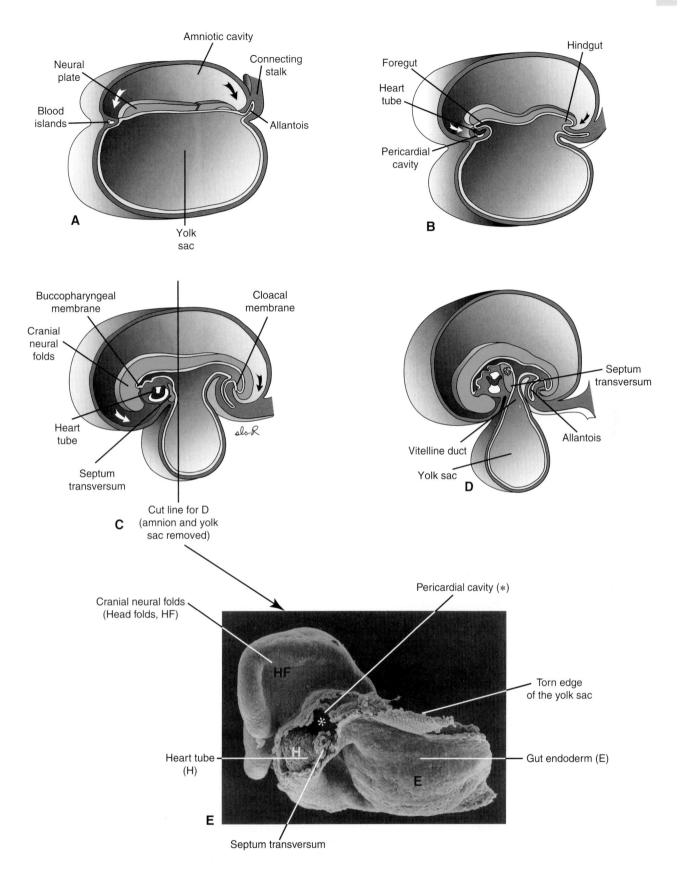

FIGURE 5.2. Lateral folding of the embryonic disc creates the heart tube by fusion, and cephalic folding brings the tube into the thoracic region (**A–D**). This cephalic fold is formed primarily by rapid growth of the cranial neural folds (head folds) derived from the neural plate (**C** and **E**). The pericardial cavity is represented by the space (intraembryonic cavity) between splanchnic and somatic layers of lateral plate mesoderm (**B** and **E**; see Figs. 3.6 and 3.7). Because the heart tube itself develops from splanchnic mesoderm lining this cavity, the tube bulges into the **pericardial cavity** from its inception (**C**). The heart and pericardial sac also are adjacent to a section of mesoderm called the **septum transversum** that ultimately forms the **central tendon of the diaphragm** (**C** and **E**; see Fig. 3.6). This relation explains why the pericardial sac is anchored to the diaphragm.

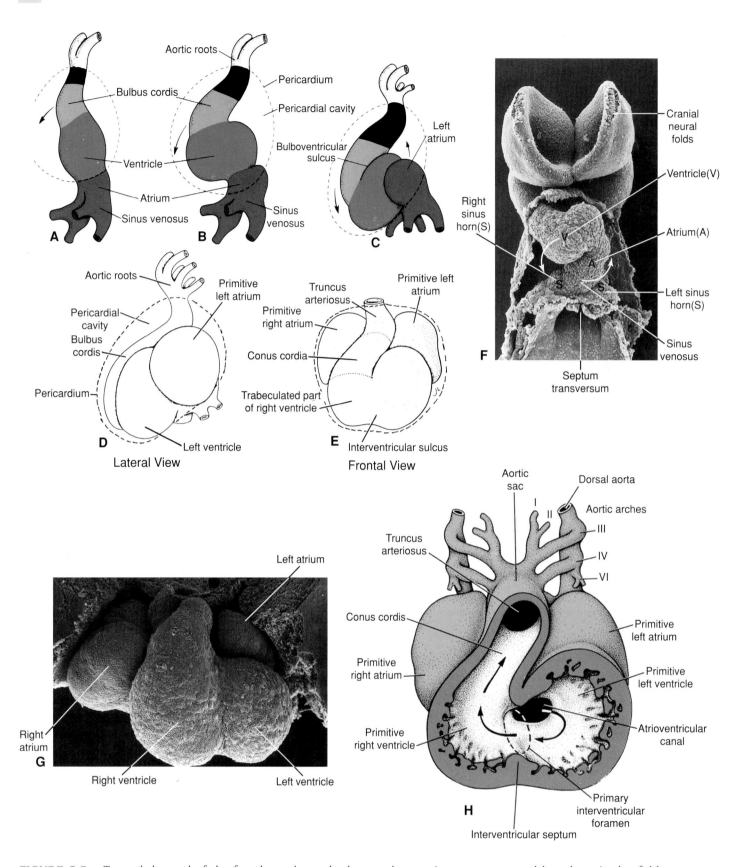

FIGURE 5.3. Toward the end of the fourth week, as the heart tube continues to grow and lengthen, it also folds upon itself, a process called "**looping**." During looping, the ventricular region grows anteriorly, caudally, and to the right; while the atrial region grows posteriorly, cranially, and to the left (**A–F**; see arrows in **F**). This repositioning and folding creates a more "typical" external appearance for the cardiac primordia, with the future atria, ventricles, and outflow tracts (conus cordis and truncus arteriosus) apparent by the end of the fourth week (**G** and **H**). However, internally there are no subdivisions between these chambers because septa partitioning them have not yet formed (**H**). **Dextrocardia** (right-sided heart) results when looping occurs in the opposite direction.

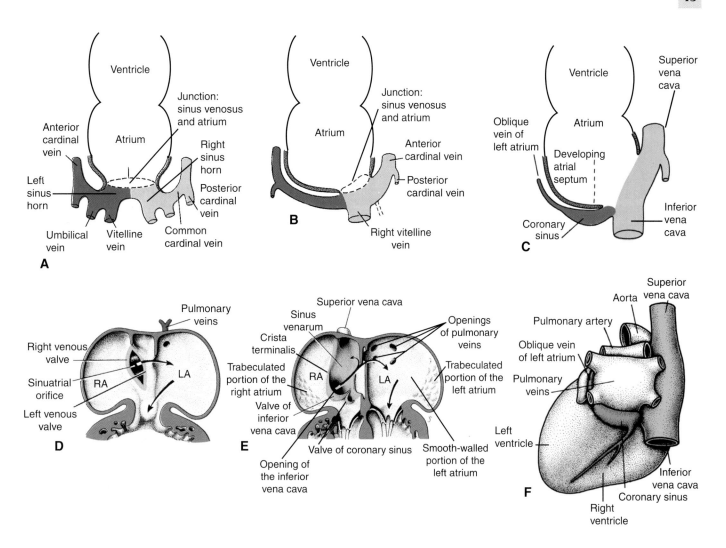

FIGURE 5.4. While looping is occurring, the heart chambers are expanding and differentiating, especially in the atrial region. Initially, the **common atrium** communicates with the **sinus venosus**, which has **left and right horns**. Each of these horns receives three vessels: (1) a **vitelline vein** coming from the yolk sac; (2) an **umbilical vein** from the placenta; and (3) a **common cardinal vein**, which receives the **anterior** and **posterior cardinal veins** draining the head and body of the embryo, respectively (**A**; see also Fig. 5.10A). As development continues, use of veins on the left side of the embryo diminishes, and definitive channels shift to the right (see Fig. 5.13). Simultaneously, the atrial region enlarges and incorporates the sinus venosus into itself, and, because of the shift in venous flow from left to right, this incorporation is directed toward the right atrium (**B–D**). Eventually, the entire region of the sinus venosus and right sinus horn becomes part of the future right atrium (**D**), and all that remains on the left is part of the left sinus horn, which forms the **coronary sinus** and **oblique vein of Marshal** (**C** and **F**). In the right atrium, the incorporated sinus venosus forms the **smooth-walled (sinus venarum) portion** of this structure, with a ridge, the **crista terminalis**, representing the boundary between the original portion of the right atrium that is trabeculated and the part derived from the sinus venosus (**E**). Early in development, incorporation of the sinus region creates a set of valves around the opening into the right atrium (**D**). The left-hand portion of these valves disappears, while the right-hand side develops into the **valve of the coronary sinus** and the **valve of the inferior vena cava** (**E**). The valve of the inferior vena cava is important because it helps direct blood returning from this vessel across the opening (**foramen ovale**) in the interatrial septum during fetal life (**E**; see Fig. 5.5B). Expansion of the left atrium also occurs, but in a different manner from the right. This chamber sprouts a vessel from its posterior wall, the **pulmonary vein** (**D**). This vessel branches, forms connections with the lungs, and establishes the system of pulmonary veins. As the primitive left atrium grows, it incorporates the root of the original vessel and the initial part of its first four branches. Thus, the smooth-walled part of the left atrium is derived from the initial segments of the pulmonary vein and its branches, thereby accounting for the four openings of these vessels into this chamber (**D–F**).

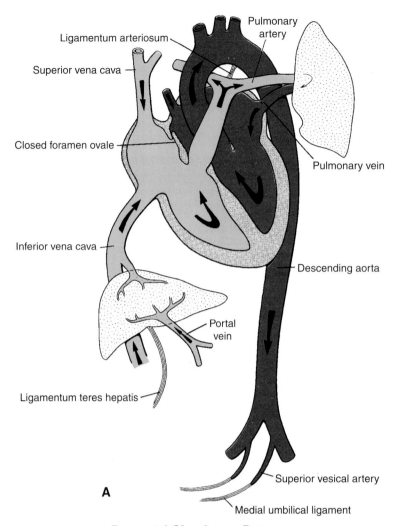

Postnatal Circulatory Pattern

FIGURE 5.5. To understand the process of septation of the heart into its four chambers and two outflow tracts, a knowledge of the circulatory patterns during postnatal versus fetal life is necessary. After birth, venous blood from the head and the rest of the body returns to the right atrium via the superior and inferior vena cavae, respectively. Blood then flows to the right ventricle, to the pulmonary trunk, to the lungs, back through the pulmonary veins to the left atrium, to the left ventricle and out the aorta to all parts of the body (**A**). However, during fetal life, the lungs are not functional, and oxygenated blood returns from the placenta through the umbilical vein to the inferior vena cava to the right atrium (**B**). From here this blood must enter the left side of the heart and bypass the nonfunctioning lungs so that it can enter the aorta to provide oxygen and nutrients to all parts of the body. Therefore, a system must develop that permits this transfer from right atrium to left during fetal life, but reverses it to the postnatal configuration at birth. This phenomenon is accomplished by constructing a unidirectional flutter valve in the interatrial septum that allows most of the blood returning to the right atrium from the inferior vena cava to "shunt" across into the left atrium (**B**) where it can enter the left ventricle and thence the aorta. This passageway is called the **foramen ovale** (**B**). After birth, the lungs inflate, pulmonary circulation is established, and blood returns from the lungs to the left atrium. Pressure in this chamber becomes greater than in the right, forcing the valve to close. Later, the valve seals itself with fibrous tissue and closure becomes permanent. (continued)

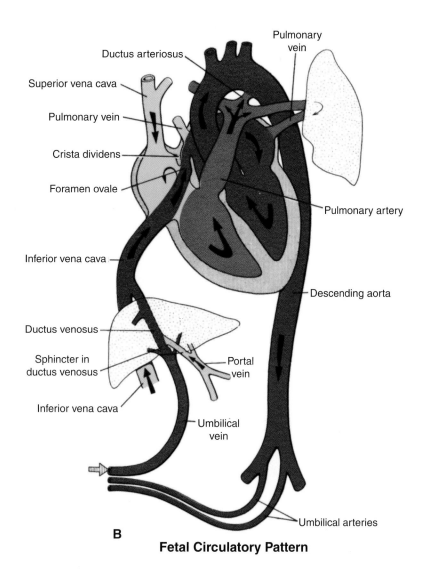

Fetal Circulatory Pattern

FIGURE 5.5. (*Continued*) In addition to this interatrial shunt, two other shunts are constructed in the fetal circulation (**B**). The **ductus venosus** connects the umbilical vein to the inferior vena cava, thereby bypassing the liver. Because the liver functions as an hematopoietic (blood-forming) organ during fetal life, it is not used for processing nutrients from the gut via the portal venous system as it will do postnatally. In addition to bypassing the liver, the ductus venosus regulates blood flow from the placenta to the heart and prevents sudden surges in blood volume that might result from increased intra-abdominal pressure in the mother, such as when she coughs or has a bowel movement. The vessel closes upon clamping of the umbilical cord at birth and later forms a fibrous cord, the **ligamentum venosum**. Another shunt, the **ductus arteriosus**, connects the pulmonary trunk with the aorta. The shunt allows most of the blood pumped into the pulmonary artery by the right ventricle to bypass the lungs. Most of this blood is derived from that returning to the right atrium from the superior vena cava. As it enters the right atrium, there is some mixing with blood arriving via the inferior vena cava (oxygenated blood from the placenta), but for the most part these two streams are kept separate by a valve on the inferior vena cava at its junction with the atrium that directs blood arriving from the inferior vena cava toward the left atrium across the foramen ovale. At birth, the ductus arteriosus also closes, forming the **ligamentum arteriosum**. The signal causing closure is **bradykinin**, a substance released by the lungs when they inflate that interacts with receptors on smooth muscle cells surrounding the ductus, causing their contraction and closure of this shunt.

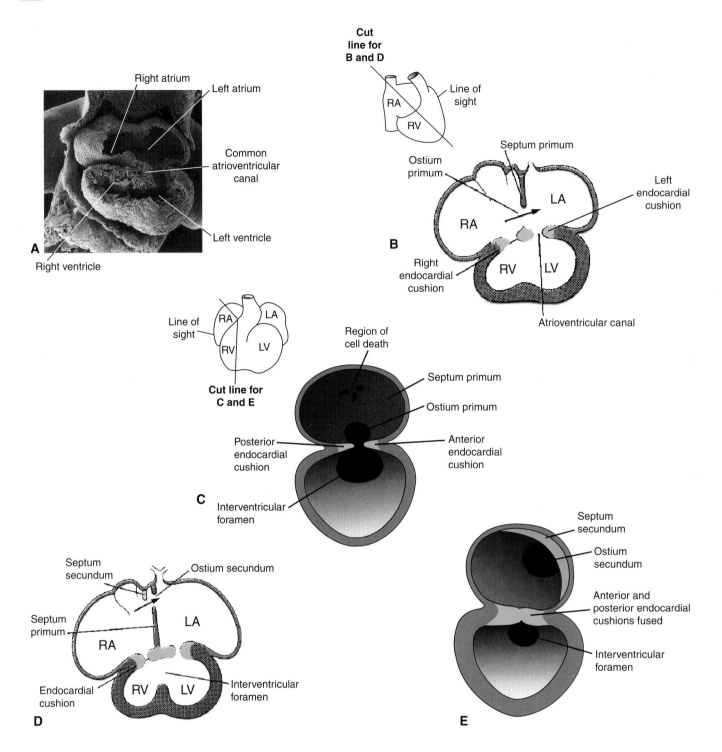

FIGURE 5.6. As discussed previously, heart looping and differential growth create the more familiar external appearance of the heart and set the stage for its septation into four chambers and two outflow tracts. Before septation occurs, however, all of the future chambers communicate with each other, and there is a single **atrioventricular canal** linking the common atrium with the ventricle (**A** and **B**). Septation occurs simultaneously during the fifth and sixth weeks in all regions. However, the **atrial septum** develops in such a way that blood returning from the placenta via the inferior vena cava can be shunted over to the left atrium (**B**). Thus, in the atria, two septa grow down from the roof to form an overlapping valve (**B–G**). The **first septum (septum primum)** grows downward toward **endocardial cushions** that surround the atrioventricular canal (**B** and **C**). There are four of these cushions (**B** and **C**). The anterior (inferior) and posterior (superior) cushions grow toward each other and fuse in the midline, thereby separating the original atrioventricular canal into right and left openings (**C** and **E**). Their fusion also creates a platform for contact with the septum primum. Before this contact is made, the opening between the septum primum and the fused cushions is called the **ostium (opening) primum** (**B**). As this opening is being eliminated by fusion of the septum primum with the atrioventricular endocardial cushions, a **second opening (ostium secundum)** is created near the top of the septum primum by a process of programmed cell death (apoptosis; **C–E**). Creation of the ostium secundum is essential to maintain blood flow from the right atrium to the left.   (continued)

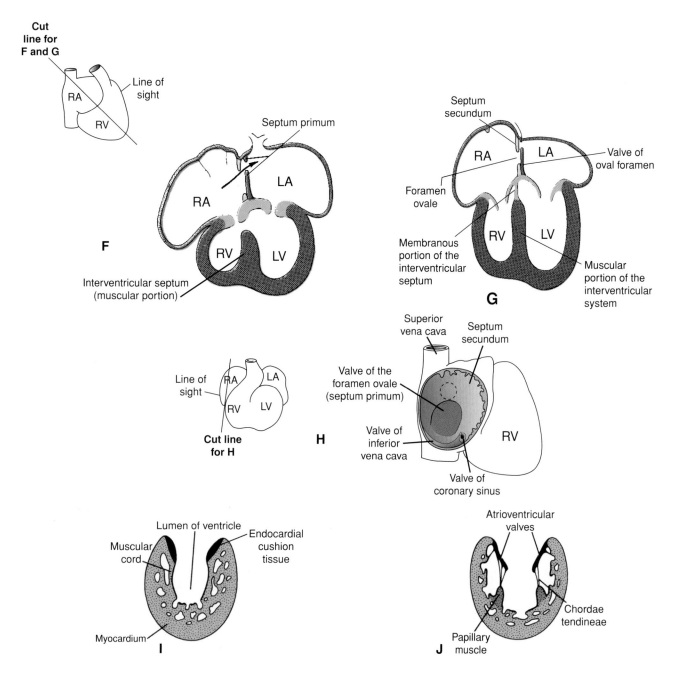

FIGURE 5.6. *(Continued)* Next, a **second septum (septum secundum)** grows from the atrial roof to the right of the septum primum toward the platform created by fusion of the endocardial cushions (**D** and **E**). However, it never forms a complete septum, but instead maintains an opening (**D–H**). In this manner, an oblique valve-covered opening, the **foramen ovale (oval foramen)**, is established between the atria. The valve is formed by the septum primum as it overlaps the septum secundum and covers the foramen ovale (**G** and **H**). In the fetus, this valve is deflected toward the left, allowing oxygenated blood from the right atrium to flow through the foramen ovale. At birth, the valve is pressed against the septum secundum, and closure of the interatrial septum is completed. Septum formation in the ventricles is simpler (**F** and **G**). A **muscular portion** forms from expansion of the ventricles laterally and proliferation of muscular tissue. Septation is completed by growth of endocardial cushion tissue downward to fuse with the muscular portion. Thus, the top of the ventricular septum is derived from endocardial cushion tissue and is **membranous**, not muscular (**G**). Continued differentiation of endocardial tissue around the atrioventricular canal produces the **tricuspid** and **bicuspid (mitral) valves** in the right and left atrioventricular canals, respectively (**G**). Muscular cords form attachments to the valves and differentiate into the **chordae tendineae** and **papillary muscles** (**I** and **J**). These attachments keep the valve leaflets from everting into the atria when the ventricles contract. LA, left atrium; LV, left ventricle; RA, right atrium; RV, right ventricle.

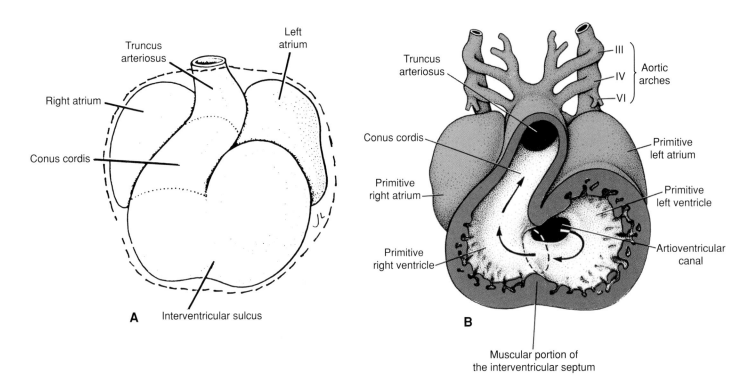

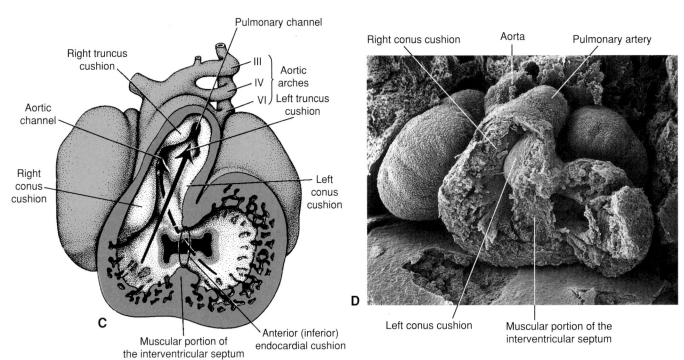

FIGURE 5.7. The **outflow tract** also is partitioned by endocardial-like cushion tissue into the **pulmonary** and **aortic trunks**. The tract consists of the **conus cordis** and **truncus arteriosus** (**A** and **B**), and **endocardial cushion tissue** forms along the sides of each of these regions (**C** and **D**). Interestingly, **neural crest cells** migrate from neural folds in the hindbrain to form these cushions. (continued)

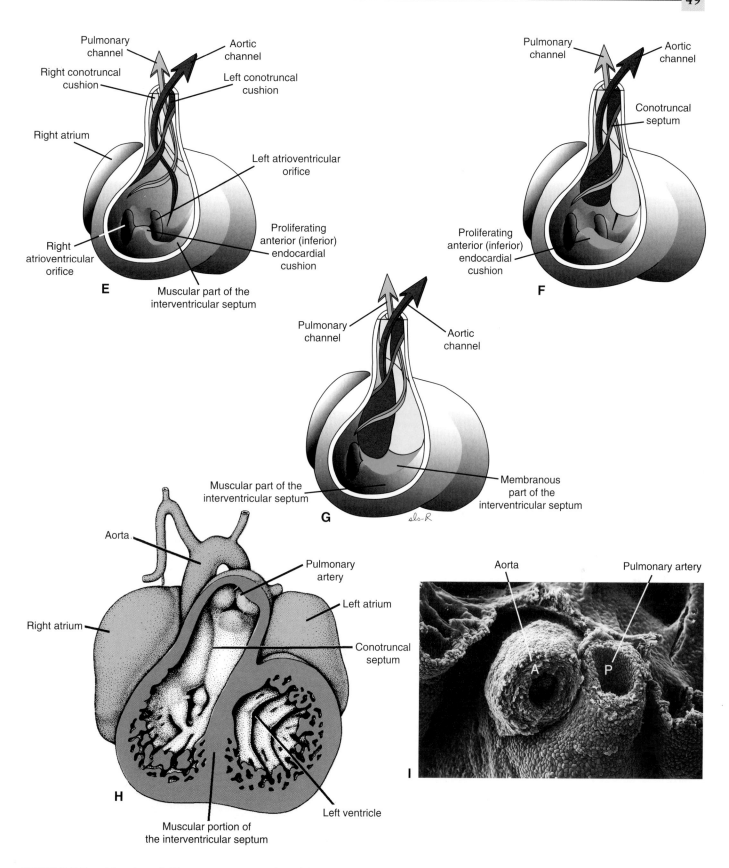

FIGURE 5.7. *(Continued)* These **conotruncal cushions** grow toward the midline and fuse, spiraling 180 degrees as they do so (**C** and **E–H**). They also grow downward and fuse with endocardial cushion tissue, which contributes to the membranous portion of the interventricular septum (**E–G**; see Fig. 5.6G). Their spiral course accounts for the intertwining path of the pulmonary and aortic vessels as they leave the heart (**I**) and also places the pulmonary opening in the right ventricle and the aortic opening in the left ventricle (**E–G**).

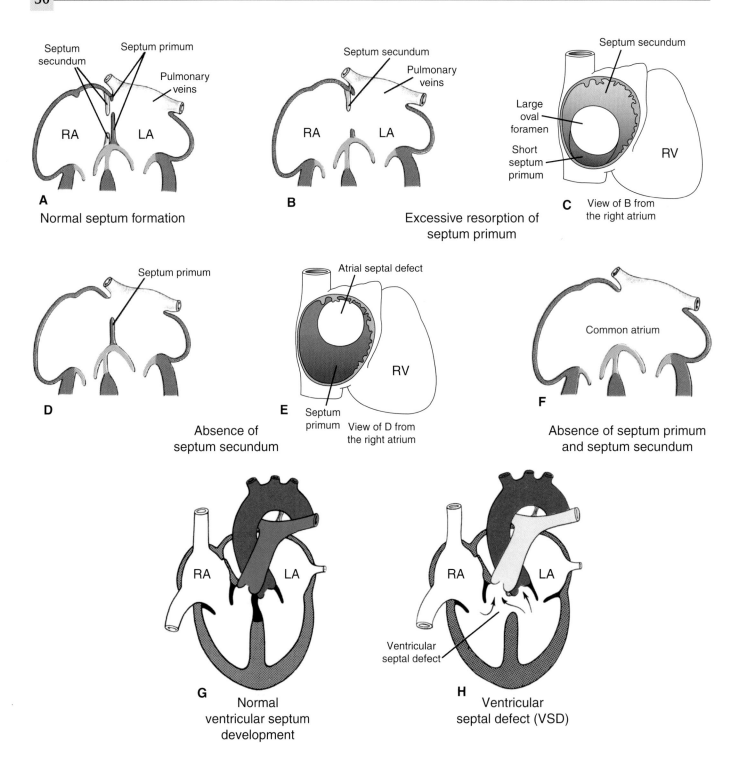

FIGURE 5.8. Because of the complexity of cardiac development, it is not surprising that heart malformations are the most common type of birth defect. **Atrial septal defects (ASDs)** occur in 6 of every 10,000 births and may be due to excessive cell death in the septum primum, causing an enlarged ostium secundum (**A–C**); incomplete development of the septum secundum (**D** and **E**); or absence of both septa (common atrium; **F**). Many other heart defects are caused by abnormalities of endocardial cushion tissue, which plays such a key role in septation. Thus, failure of proliferation of the atrioventricular cushions to form the membranous portion of the interventricular septum results in a **ventricular septal defect (VSD)**, the most common heart malformation, which is seen in 12 of every 10,000 births (**G** and **H**). LA, left atrium; RA, right atrium; RV, right ventricle.

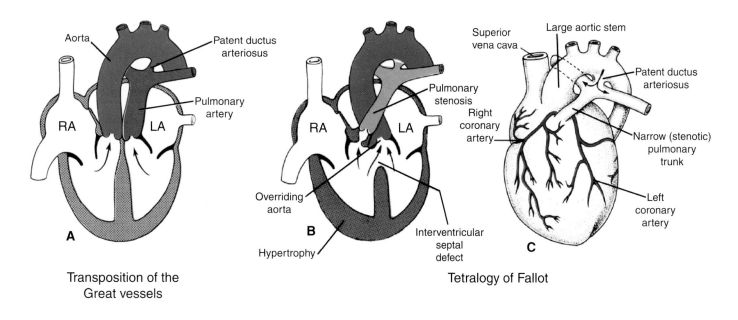

Transposition of the
Great vessels

Tetralogy of Fallot

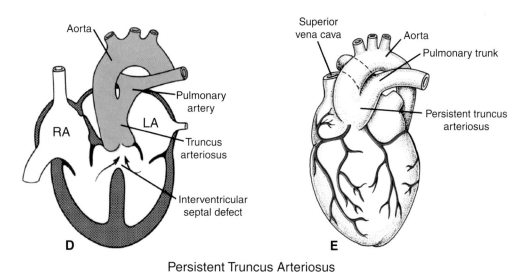

Persistent Truncus Arteriosus

FIGURE 5.9. **Endocardial-like cushions** in the **conotruncal region** also may develop abnormally, resulting in **outflow tract defects**. **Transposition of the great vessels** (seen in 5 of every 10,000 births), with the aorta originating from the right ventricle and the pulmonary trunk from the left, occurs when this septum fails to spiral and instead grows straight downward (**A**). Anterior displacement of the septum results in a constellation of four heart abnormalities called the **tetralogy of Fallot** (**B** and **C**). In this situation, anterior positioning of this septum causes (1) narrowing (stenosis) of the pulmonary trunk; (2) a concomitant enlargement of the aorta, such that this vessel is positioned above the ventricular septum (i.e., an overriding aorta); (3) a VSD, because the cushions in the conus fail to join those around the atrioventricular canal; and (4) hypertrophy (enlargement) of the right ventricle due to an increased work load caused by shunting of blood across the VSD and stenosis (narrowing) of the pulmonary trunk. Yet another defect in this region, called **persistent truncus arteriosus** (seen in 1 in every 10,000 births), occurs if the cushions fail to form at all (**D** and **E**). This defect is always accompanied by a VSD because no link is made between conotruncal cushions and endocardial cushions in the atrioventricular region. Importantly, **neural crest cells**, derived from neuroepithelial cells in the neural folds, contribute to formation of the conotruncal cushions. Since populations of these cells also form bones and connective tissue in the face (see Fig. 4.3A), it is not surprising that in many cases craniofacial and heart defects occur together. Neural crest cells are particularly sensitive to environmental insults and genetic aberrations, which may account for the high incidence of defects involving the heart and face. LA, left atrium; RA, right atrium.

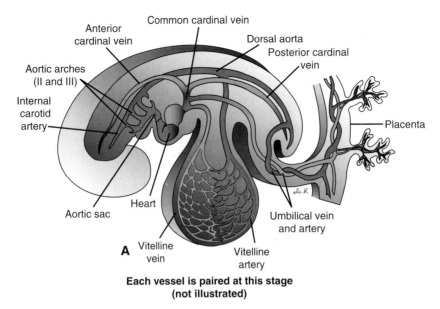

Each vessel is paired at this stage
(not illustrated)

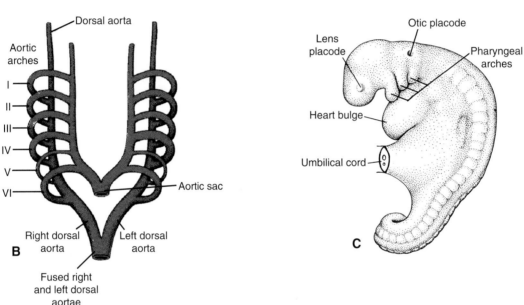

FIGURE 5.10. Vascular development occurs by two methods: (1) **vasculogenesis**, whereby clusters of cells aggregate to form blood islands that later coalesce into vessels; and (2) **angiogenesis**, where new vessels sprout from existing ones. By the beginning of the fifth week, a system of arteries and veins, in which each vessel is paired, has been established to serve the head and body of the embryo, the yolk sac, and the developing placenta (**A**). Thus, a paired series of **aortic arches** and **dorsal aortae** supply the head and body of the embryo, while paired **anterior** and **posterior cardinal veins** provide venous drainage. Paired **vitelline arteries** and paired **vitelline veins** serve the yolk sac and paired **umbilical arteries** and **veins** carry blood to and from the placenta. In the fifth week, these vascular patterns begin to be reconfigured into the adult system by fusion, sprouting of new vessels, or regression of original vessels. As these changes take place, definitive arterial vessels tend to form on the left side of the body; whereas those of veins form on the right. For example, although the original dorsal aortic vessels are paired, those supplying the body fuse into a single vessel, the descending aorta, lying to the left of the midline (**B** and **E**). Similarly, rearrangement of the venous pattern results in the superior and inferior vena cavae being positioned to the right (see Fig. 5.13F and G). Because of this reorganization, many anomalies occur, particularly in veins, but most are of no major consequence. Arteries in the head and neck form a series of arches, the **aortic arches**, on either side of the pharynx (**A** and **B**). These vessels arise from an extension of the outflow tract of the heart called the aortic sac and form a series of six pairs that connect to the dorsal aortae (the fifth is rudimentary or never forms; **A** and **B**). Each vessel courses in the core of a **pharyngeal arch**, structures analogous to the gills of a fish (**C**; see Fig. 8.1). (continued)

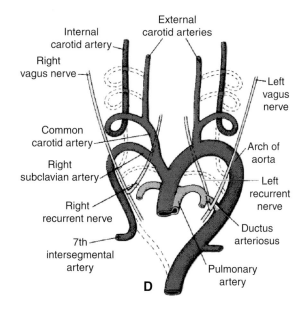

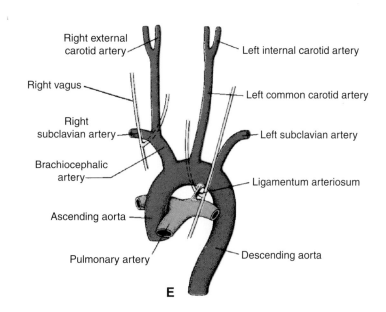

FIGURE 5.10. (*Continued*) Aortic arch vessels appear in cranial to caudal sequence, are not all present simultaneously, and undergo a significant amount of remodeling (**D** and **E**). The first and second vessels largely disappear (dotted lines in **D** represent vessels from the original aortic arch pattern [**B**] that regress), leaving only the **maxillary** (first arch) and **stapedial** and **hyoid** (second arch) arteries. The third, fourth, and sixth arches form the largest vessels. The third forms the common **carotid arteries** and the initial segments of the **internal carotid arteries**. The remainder of the internal carotid arteries form from the dorsal aorta (**B** and **D**), while the **external carotid arteries** arise as sprouts from the common carotid arteries. The fourth arch on the left forms the **aortic arch** between the common carotid and subclavian arteries. The proximal part of the aorta and the **brachiocephalic artery** on the right are derived from the right and left horns of the aortic sac, respectively. Also on the right, the fourth arch forms the proximal segment of the **subclavian artery** (**D** and **E**). The sixth arch sprouts branches from its proximal segments that form the **pulmonary arteries** to the lungs. As these connections are established, the distal portion of the sixth arch on the right degenerates, but on the left it remains to form the **ductus arteriosus** (**D**), connecting the pulmonary trunk to the descending aorta so that most of the blood from the right ventricle bypasses the lungs during fetal life. At birth, the ductus closes and becomes the **ligamentum arteriosum** (**E**). In addition to an aortic arch artery, each pharyngeal arch also has its own cranial nerve (see Fig. 8.1). The nerve to the sixth arch is the recurrent laryngeal branch of the vagus nerve (cranial nerve X). Because a portion of the sixth arch on the right degenerates (**D**), this nerve "slips up" to the level of the right subclavian artery (**D** and **E**). However, on the left it remains "hooked" around the ductus arteriosus (ligamentum arteriosum; **E**) because this portion of the sixth arch does not regress.

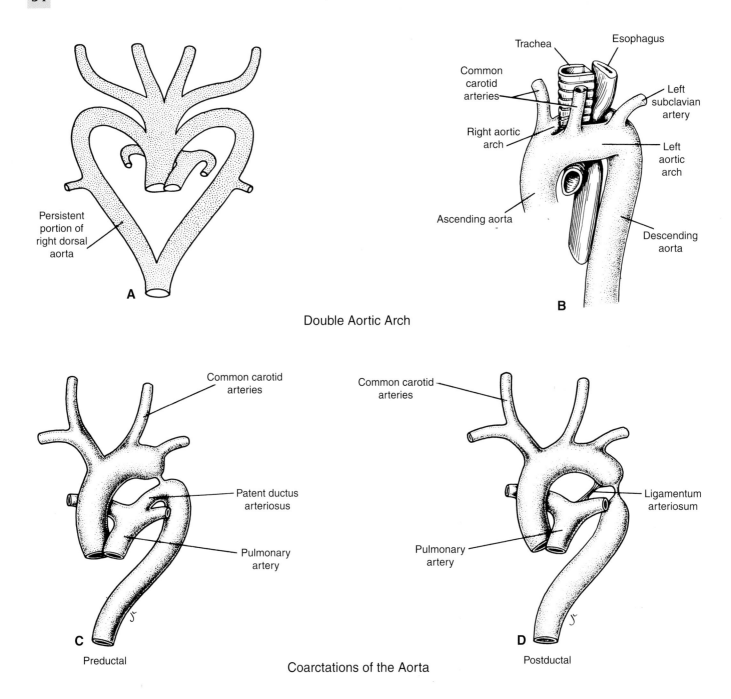

Double Aortic Arch

Coarctations of the Aorta

FIGURE 5.11.   Abnormalities in the aortic arch system are rare, but may occur if a vessel that is supposed to regress remains intact or extra parts of vessels are lost. For example, if the distal portion of the right fourth aortic arch remains, then a **double-arched aorta** is formed (**A**; see also **B** and **D**). Because these arches pass around both sides of the trachea and esophagus, difficulties with swallowing may ensue (**B**). Another serious vessel defect that may occur is **coarctation of the aorta**, either preductal (proximal to the entrance of the ductus arteriosus; **C**) or postductal (distal to the junction of the ductus; **D**). The cause is not known, but may be related to abnormalities in receptor ligand signaling that normally initiate closure of the ductus arteriosus at birth. The postductal defect is more common and is circumvented by collateral circulation through the internal thoracic and intercostal arteries. Sometimes the ductus fails to close, resulting in a **patent ductus arteriosus** (seen in 8 per 10,000 births).

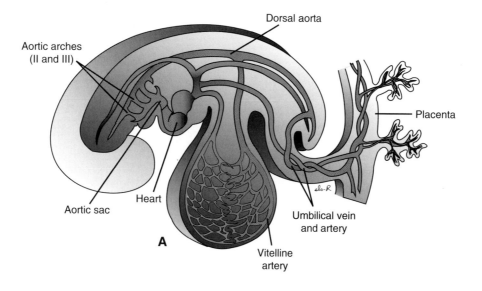

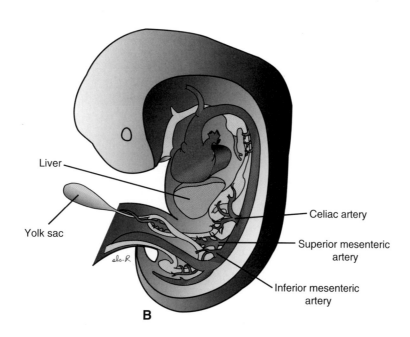

FIGURE 5.12.   Paired **vitelline arteries** supply the yolk sac (**A**). As the embryo folds cephalocaudally and laterally to form the gut tube and narrow the connection of the yolk sac to a small opening at the umbilicus (see Fig. 3.5), these arteries are redirected to supply various regions of the gut tube. Thus, the **celiac artery** forms from more cranially placed vitelline vessels and serves the **foregut**; middle-placed vessels form the **superior mesenteric artery** supplying the **midgut**; and distal vessels form the **inferior mesenteric artery** supplying the **hindgut** (**B**). **Umbilical arteries** are branches of the paired dorsal aortae (**A**). Later, when the lower limbs develop, they shift position to arise from the common iliac arteries. After birth, proximal segments of the umbilical arteries persist as the **internal iliac** and **superior vesical arteries**. Distal portions are obliterated to form the **medial umbilical ligaments**.

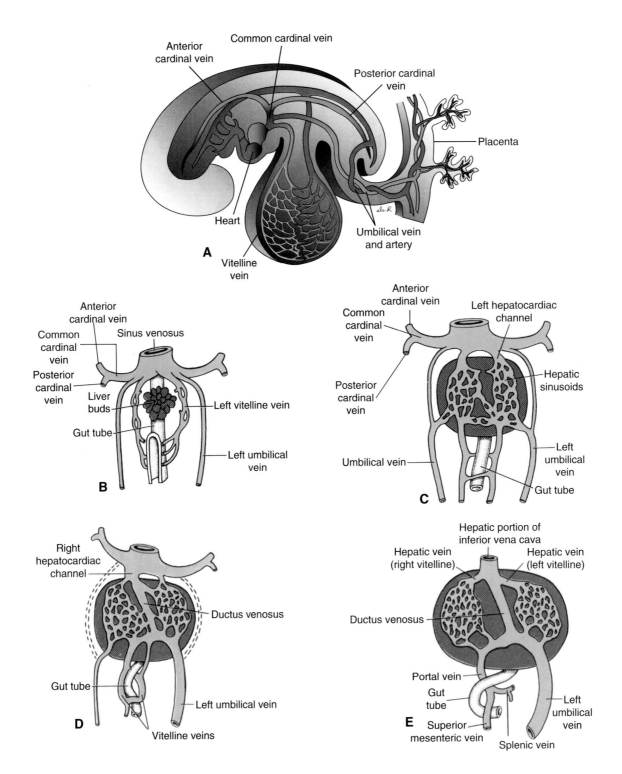

FIGURE 5.13. Initially, three major sets of paired veins develop (**A**): (1) **vitelline (yolk sac) veins,** which drain the yolk sac; (2) **umbilical veins,** which drain the placenta; and (3) **cardinal veins,** which drain the body. Changes in the vitelline veins occur as cephalocaudal and lateral folding of the embryo closes the gut tube (see Fig. 3.5), reducing the opening of the yolk sac to a narrow outlet at the umbilicus. As folding occurs, the vitelline veins assume more and more of the drainage for the gut tube (**A** and **B**) and eventually reorganize to form the **portal system of veins** draining the gut from the caudal end of the esophagus to the middle of the rectum (**C–E**). In addition, because the liver grows out from the gut tube into the region served by vitelline veins, these veins form the **hepatic sinusoids** and **hepatic veins** (**B** and **C**). Umbilical veins also undergo major alterations (**A–D**). The right is lost completely, as is the proximal segment of the left (**C** and **D**). The distal segment of the left enlarges and becomes the **definitive umbilical vein** (**D** and **E**). It also forms a connection with a channel called the **ductus venosus,** which empties into the inferior vena cava (**D** and **E**). The ductus itself forms from a coalescence of small channels derived from the hepatic sinusoids (vitelline veins; **C** and **D**) and serves to bypass the liver for blood coming from the placenta via the umbilical vein. At birth, the umbilical vein and ductus venosus close and later form the **ligamentum teres hepatis (round ligament of the liver)** and the **ligamentum venosum,** respectively. *(continued)*

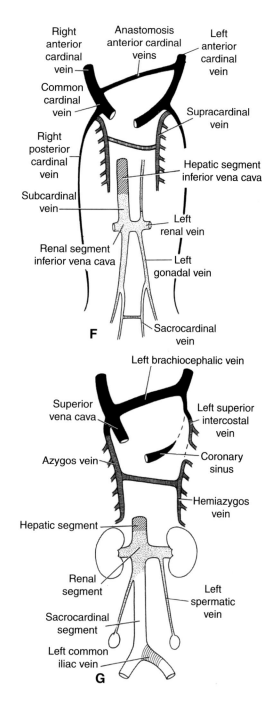

FIGURE 5.13. (*Continued*) Paired **cardinal veins** drain the body during early embryonic development (through the 4th week). **Anterior cardinal veins** drain the head and upper limb buds, while **posterior cardinal veins** drain the rest of the body (**A**). Both the anterior and posterior veins on each side unite at the **common cardinal veins** that flow into the **sinus venosus** and ultimately into the common atrium (**A** and **B**). During the 5th through 7th weeks, changes occur in this pattern as the embryo and its organ systems develop (**F**). For the most part, anterior cardinal veins are retained. An anastomosis between the two forms the **left brachiocephalic vein**, and anterior segments from both form the **jugular system** for the head and neck (**F** and **G**). Most of the posterior segment on the left disappears except for that forming the left superior intercostal vein, whereas the right posterior segment forms the **superior vena cava** (**F** and **G**). In contrast to the anterior cardinal system, most of the posterior system disappears as various organs develop and establish their own veinous drainage (**F** and **G**). For example, as the thoracic cavity and ribs develop, **supracardinal veins** differentiate and ultimately form the **azygous** (right side) and **hemiazygous** (left side) collections of veins. Similarly, when the kidneys appear, a **subcardinal system** is established that eventually creates the **gonadal veins, right and left renal veins**, and the **renal segment of the inferior vena cava**. As the abdomen, pelvis, and lower limbs develop, **sacrocardinal veins** form and later reorganize to create the lower segment of the **inferior vena cava** and proximal portion of the **iliac veins** draining the lower limbs (**F** and **G**). Note that the inferior vena cava is comprised of hepatic, renal, and abdominal segments, derived from the right vitelline, subcardinal, and sacrocardinal veins, respectively (**F** and **G**). Because of the complexity of development in the venous system, anomalies are common. Usually, however, these anomalies are not of clinical significance, except to a surgeon who is tying off vessels during an operation.

CHAPTER 6

Lungs and Gut

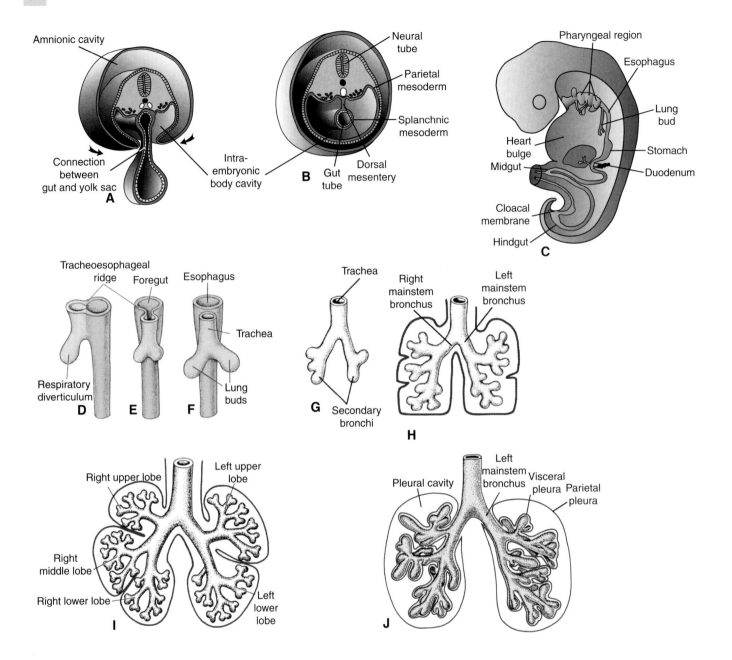

FIGURE 6.1. The **gut tube** forms when the embryo folds laterally, causing the endoderm layer of the germ disc to roll into a tube ventral to the ectoderm-derived neural tube (**A** and **B**; the embryo is a tube on top of a tube held together by mesoderm; see Fig. 3.5.). The gut tube is divided into four segments (**C**): (1) the **pharynx**, extending from the buccopharyngeal membrane to just proximal to the lung bud (described with craniofacial development; see Chapter 8); (2) the **foregut**, extending from the lung bud to the liver bud; (3) the **midgut**, extending from just caudal to the liver bud to the proximal two thirds of the transverse colon; and (4) the **hindgut**, extending from the left one third of the transverse colon to the cloacal membrane. **Endoderm** forms the epithelial lining of the gut tube, whereas muscle, connective tissue, and peritoneal components of the wall of the gut are derived from **splanchnic mesoderm**. The foregut differentiates into the esophagus, stomach, and part of the duodenum down to and including the liver bud and is unique because of its propensity to form **endodermal buds** that grow into surrounding mesoderm to become organs, including the lungs, liver, gallbladder, and pancreas. In each case, endoderm forms the functional cells of the organ (the **parenchyma**), while mesoderm forms the **connective tissue stroma**. All of the organ buds appear in the 4th week. The **lung bud (respiratory diverticulum)** arises at the cranial end of the foregut at its junction with the back of the pharynx (**C**). The bud is soon divided from the foregut by the **tracheoesophageal septum**, which forms from two **tracheoesophageal ridges**, and this septum separates the trachea anteriorly from the foregut posteriorly (**D–F**). The bud divides into **right** and **left mainstem bronchi**, and these form three **secondary bronchi** on the right and two on the left, reflecting the fact that the right lung has three lobes and the left has two (**G–I**). Secondary bronchi continue dividing into smaller and smaller channels to create the **bronchial tree** for the lobes of each lung (**I**). In fact, six additional divisions occur postnatally to complete this tree (see Table 6.1 for stages of lung development). Splanchnic mesoderm covering the lung buds (**B**) forms tracheal and bronchial cartilages and surrounding connective tissue. It also forms the **visceral pleura** covering the lungs in the **pleural cavity** (**J**; see Fig. 3.8A and B).

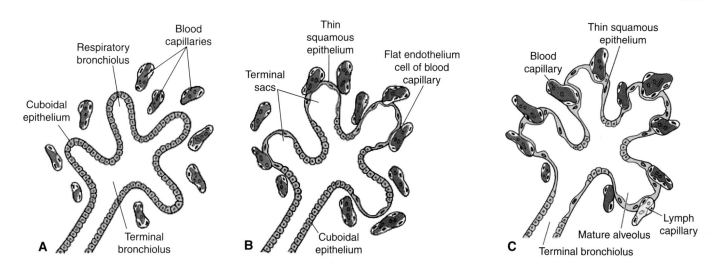

Table 6.1. **Maturation of the Lungs**

Stage	Timing	Developmental Events
Pseudoglandular	5–16 wks	Branching has continued to form terminal bronchioles. No respiratory bronchioles or alveoli are present.
Canalicular period	16–26 wks	Each terminal bronchiole divides into two or more respiratory bronchioles, which in turn divide into three to six alveolar ducts.
Terminal sac period	26 wks to birth	Terminal sacs (primitive alveoli) form, and capillaries establish close contact.
Alveolar period	8 mo (prenatally to childhood)	Mature alveoli have well-developed epithelial endothelial (capillary) contacts.

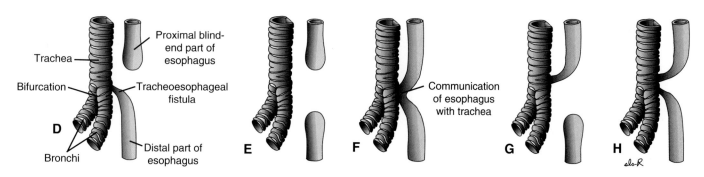

FIGURE 6.2.   Final divisions of the bronchial tree form **terminal bronchioli, respiratory bronchioli,** and **terminal sacs** that complete their differentiation by forming **alveoli (A–C)**. The many divisions of the lung buds creates an enormous surface area for gas exchange in the alveoli. Here the walls of the alveolar sacs become extremely thin and membranous and are closely apposed to a rich capillary bed (**C**). The cells that make up this network for gas exchange are **type I alveolar cells. Type II alveolar cells** do not begin development until the 6th month, are interspersed among type I cells, and produce **surfactant**, a phospholipid fluid that reduces surface tension in alveolar sacs. Without surfactant, alveoli would not be able to expand during inspiration. The necessity for surfactant explains why **premature babies** (<7 months gestation) have difficulty breathing and develop **respiratory distress syndrome (RDS)**. Artificial surfactants and corticosteroid therapy have made it possible to save babies born prior to 7 months gestation. Other lung abnormalities are rare, although occasionally ectopic lobes may arise from additional lung buds. Similarly, supernumerary lobules may form from variations in divisions of the bronchiole tree, but these usually have little significance. Of greater concern are a variety of **esophageal atresias** and **tracheoesophageal fistulas** that arise from abnormal positioning or formation of the tracheoesophageal septum (**D–H**). Five varieties of these defects occur, with 90% resulting in a blind-ending pouch in the upper esophagus combined with a tracheoesophageal fistula (**D**). Other defects, with two esophageal pouches (**E**) or a communication between the esophagus and trachea (**F**), occur equally in 4% of cases. The other two types occur with a frequency of 1% each (**G** and **H**).

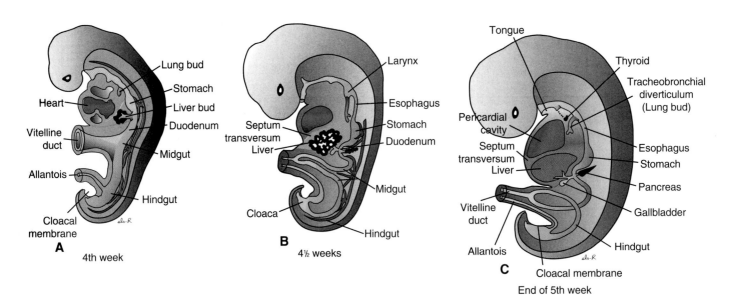

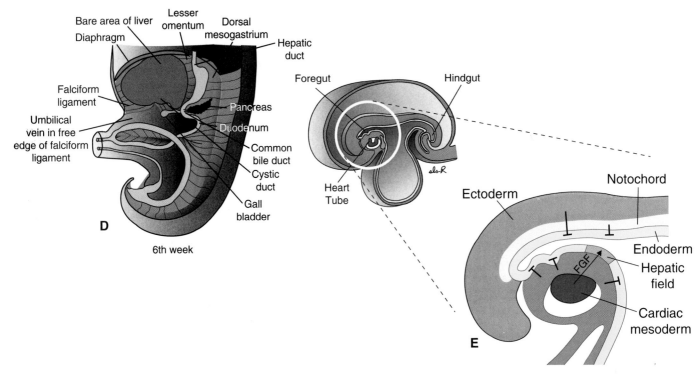

FIGURE 6.3. The **liver bud (liver diverticulum)** arises at the caudal end of the foregut and grows into mesoderm of the septum transversum (**A** and **B**). This mesoderm contributes the connective tissue for the liver, the central tendon of the diaphragm, and **ventral mesentery** of the gut (**C** and **D**) that gets separated into two parts by the liver itself: (1) the **lesser omentum**, extending from the liver to the lower esophagus, stomach, and upper duodenum; and (2) the **falciform ligament**, extending from the liver to the ventral body wall, which houses the umbilical vein in its free (caudal) border (**D**). This close association of the liver with the septum transversum is reflected by the fact that the central tendon of the diaphragm remains attached directly to the liver in the region called the **bare area of the liver** (the remainder of the liver is covered by visceral peritoneum; **D**). The proximal portion of the liver bud forms the **bile duct** and also gives rise to another bud for the **cystic duct** and **gallbladder** (**D**). During fetal life (the 10th week to the 7th month), the liver serves as the major **hematopoietic (blood-forming) organ** until bone marrow resources are established. Interestingly, the entire length of the foregut is capable of forming liver tissue, but this potential is inhibited by secreted factors arising from surrounding tissues, including the notochord and noncardiac mesoderm (**E**). However, in the liver-forming region of the foregut the inhibitory action of these factors is counteracted by FGFs secreted by adjacent cardiac mesoderm (two negatives make a plus; **E**). The net effect is upregulation of hepatocyte nuclear transcription factors *HNF3* and *HNF4* that direct endoderm cells to differentiate into liver tissue.

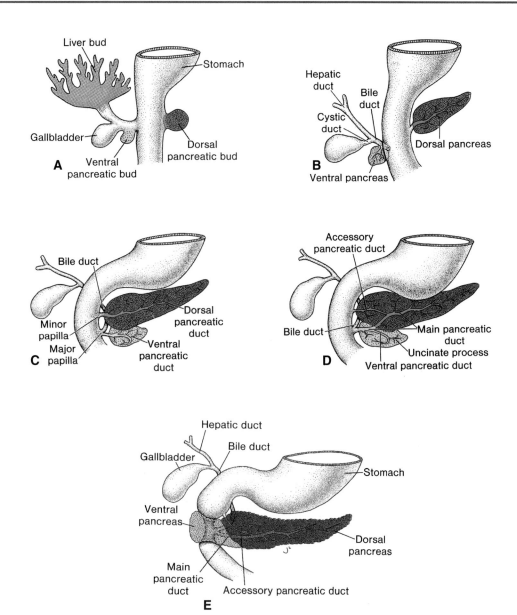

FIGURE 6.4. **Pancreas** development also begins at the distal end of the foregut (Fig. 6.3C), but in this case, two buds form on opposite sides of the gut tube: a **dorsal bud** and a **ventral bud**, the latter arising close to the liver bud (bile duct; **A** and **B**). Gradually, with differential growth of the gut tube and its rotation (see Fig. 6.6), the ventral bud moves dorsally and to the opposite side of the gut tube, until it resides just below the dorsal bud (**C** and **D**). Now the two buds fuse, and the ventral bud contributes the inferior part of the **head of the pancreas**, while the dorsal bud forms the remainder of the head and all of the **body** and **tail** (**D**). Usually the duct systems fuse as well, such that the **main pancreatic duct (of Wirsung)** is established by the distal part of the duct from the dorsal pancreatic bud and the entire duct from the ventral bud (**D**). Then, the proximal part of the duct from the dorsal pancreatic bud degenerates, although it persists as the **accessory pancreatic duct (of Santorini; D)** in about 10% of people. The main duct merges with the bile duct and enters the duodenum at the **major papilla (D)**. If present, the accessory duct enters separately at the **minor papilla**. **Pancreatic islet cells (of Langerhans)** develop at 12 weeks, and insulin secretion begins by 5 months. These cells, as well as glucagon- and somatostatin-secreting cells, are derived from gut endoderm. Occasionally, tissue from the ventral pancreatic bud grows around both sides of the duodenum, creating a condition called **annular pancreas** that may cause duodenal stenosis (**E**).

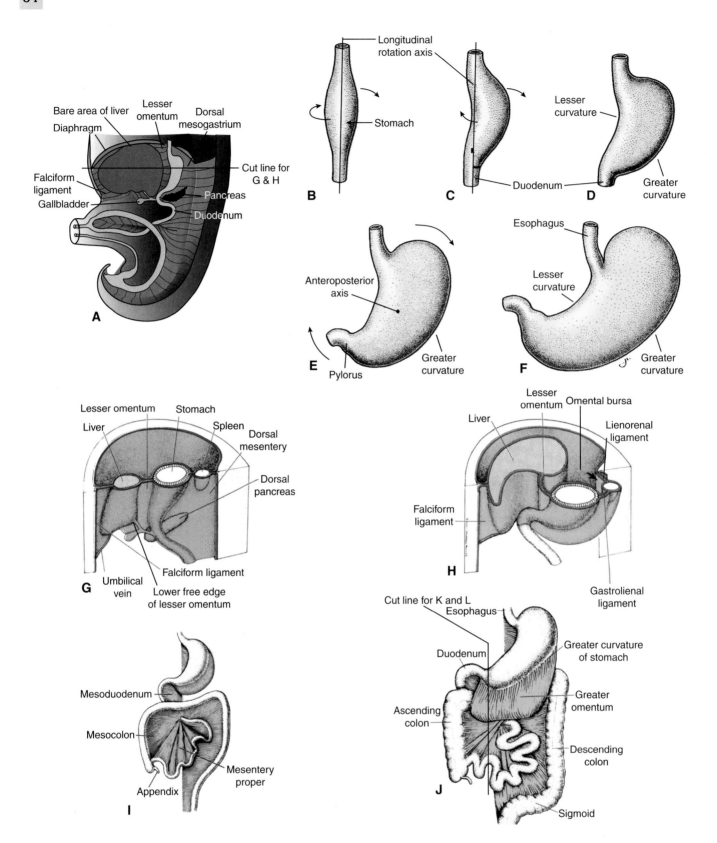

FIGURE 6.5. The **stomach** differentiates as an expansion in the foregut (**A**) and grows in such a way that its posterior border becomes larger than its anterior border, thereby creating its **greater** and **lesser curvatures** (**B–F**). The stomach also rotates 90 degrees around both its longitudinal and anterior–posterior axes, such that the original posterior border (greater curvature) becomes the left side, and the original anterior border (lesser curvature) becomes the right side (longitudinal rotation), while the original cranial and caudal ends come to lie in a more horizontal position (anteroposterior rotation; **B–F**). Rotation also changes the positions of the mesenteries attached to the stomach (**A**). Thus, the **dorsal mesentery**, attached to the greater curvature (original posterior border), gets pulled to the right and caudally, while the **ventral mesentery**, attached from the lesser curvature to the liver (the **lesser omentum**), gets pulled to the left and cranially (**G–J**). In addition, the dorsal mesentery elongates and its layers fuse to form the **greater omentum** (apron) as it hangs downward from the greater curvature to cover the intestines (**J**).

(continued)

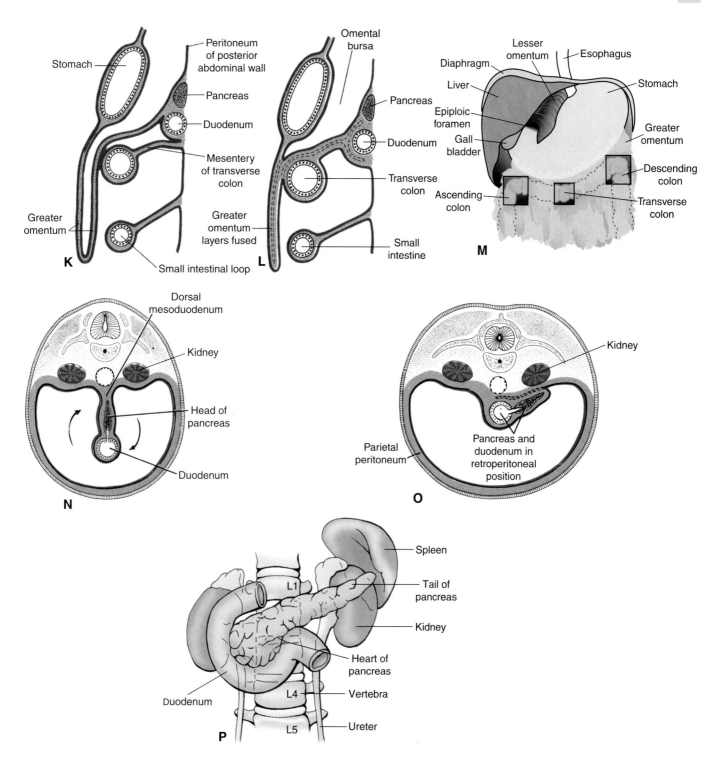

FIGURE 6.5. (*Continued*) As the greater omentum passes over the transverse colon, its posterior layer also fuses with the mesentery to this structure (the **transverse mesocolon**; **K** and **L**). The greater omentum serves as a fat storage site and is also called the "policeman" of the abdomen, because it has the capacity to move around and wall off pockets of infection. Meanwhile, ventral mesentery between the stomach and liver forms the **lesser omentum**, and its repositioning creates a space posterior to it and the stomach called the **omental bursa** or **lesser sac** (**J** and **L**). The opening into this sac is called the **epiploic foramen (of Winslow)**, and it lies posterior to the bile duct that is in the lower free edge of the lesser omentum (**G** and **M**). This opening serves as the communication between the lesser sac and the **greater sac** that includes the rest of the abdominal cavity. At the left side of the lesser sac lies the **spleen**, which differentiates directly from mesoderm of the dorsal mesentery (**G** and **H**). The **duodenum** forms from the caudal end of the foregut and from the proximal part of the midgut (**A**). Because of the stomach's rotation, the duodenum rotates to the right and twists into a "C" shape (**N–P**). It also swings to the left side of the abdominal cavity and toward the posterior wall. Here it fuses to the posterior wall (**O**) with the head of the pancreas lying in the arms of the "C" of the duodenum and tickling the spleen with its tail (**P**). Because of this fusion to the posterior wall, both the pancreas and duodenum (except its caudal end) become **retroperitoneal** and lie along the posterior aspect of the omental bursa (**L**). Thus a finger inserted into the epiploic foramen (**M**) would feel the common bile duct (and the hepatic artery and portal vein, which, with the bile duct, make up the **portal triad**) anteriorly; the pancreas posteriorly; and the spleen distal to the fingertip.

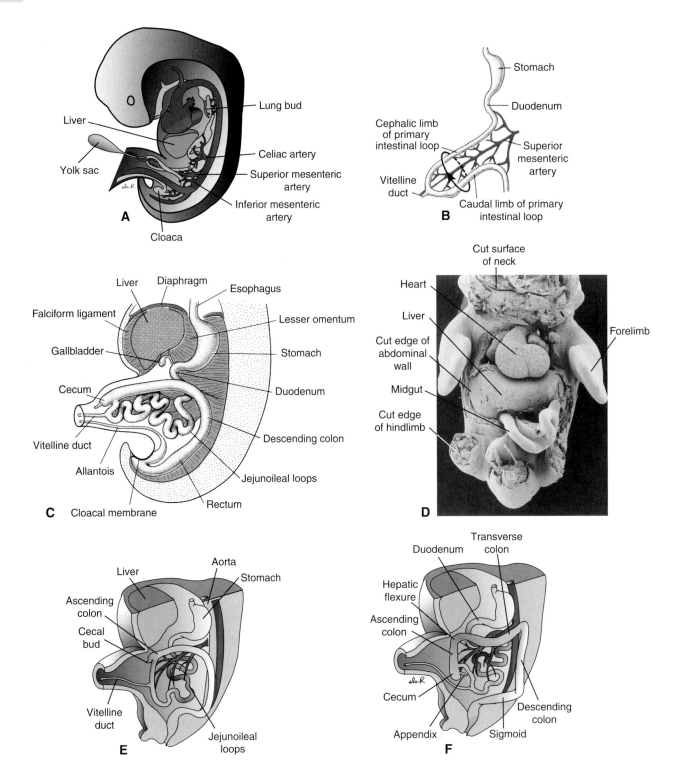

FIGURE 6.6. The **midgut** lengthens tremendously and differentiates into part of the duodenum, the small intestine (jejunum and ileum), and the appendix, cecum, ascending colon, and right two thirds of the transverse colon. As it grows, it forms the **primary intestinal loop**, which has the **superior mesenteric artery** as its axis and is connected to the yolk sac by the vitelline duct (**A**). Once formed, the primary loop rotates 270 degrees counterclockwise when viewed from the front of the embryo (**B**). The first 90-degree rotation occurs while the loop is lengthening inside the body cavity during the 5th week. Soon, however, the intestines cannot be contained within the abdominal cavity, in part because of the amount of growth of this portion of the gut compared to that of the cavity, but also because the liver occupies much of the intraabdominal space in its role as the hematopoietic organ. Therefore, in the 6th week, the loops of bowel herniate into the umbilical cord, a phenomenon called **physiological umbilical herniation** (**C** and **D**). Here the loops remain and grow until the 10th week, when they begin to return as the abdominal cavity expands. As they return, they complete another 180 degrees of rotation and settle more toward the right side (**E** and **F**). In this position, the ascending colon fuses to the posterior abdominal wall and becomes retroperitoneal, as does most of the descending colon. The remainder of the midgut derivatives retain their mesenteries.

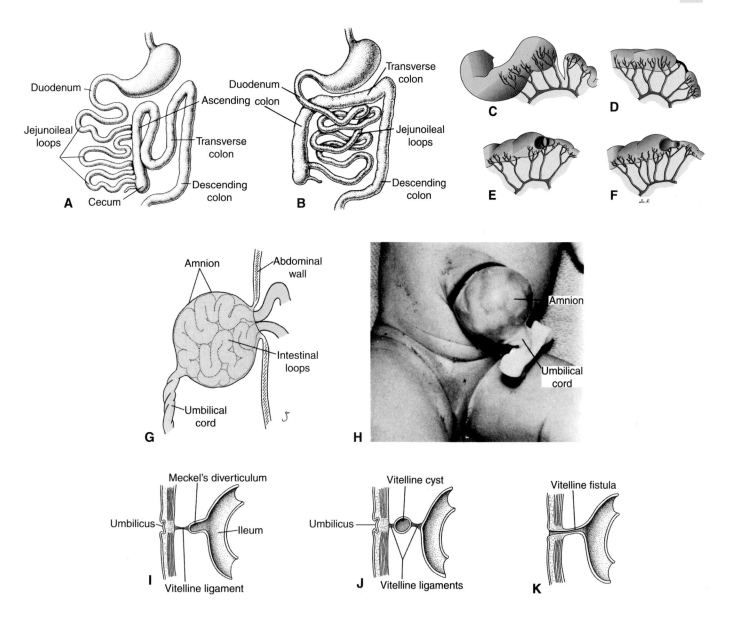

FIGURE 6.7. Several birth defects may involve the midgut. Sometimes rotation does not occur properly, resulting in abnormal positioning of the intestines. For example, if rotation only progresses 90 degrees instead of 270 degrees, then the colon and cecum are the first to return, and they settle on the left instead of the right (**A**). If rotation is reversed and occurs 90 degrees in a clockwise instead of a counterclockwise direction, then the transverse colon passes posterior to the duodenum (**B**). These rotation abnormalities may cause no observable problems, but often lead to twisting (**volvulus**) of the gut around itself, resulting in a compromised blood supply to the affected region. Disruption of vascular supply (by "**vascular accidents**") also can lead to bowel **atresias** and **stenoses**. The most common outcome (50%) results in two discontinuous bowel segments (**C**). Less often—each is seen in 20% of this group—a strand of fibrous tissue joins two affected segments (**D**) or the region is narrowed (stenosed) and contains a thin diaphragm (**E**). In 5% of cases there is a simple stenosis with no diaphragm (**F**). The origin of these vascular accidents is not known, but may involve thromboses or agenesis of vessels. **Omphalocele** is a more common birth defect, occurring in 2.5 per 10,000 births, involving the midgut. It arises when intestinal loops fail to return to the abdominal cavity following physiological umbilical herniation (**G** and **H**). Once failure to return occurs, the loops cannot simply be pushed back in, because the abdominal cavity is too small. Therefore, a "silo" is built around the area and the tube is squeezed slowly over several days from the top (like a tube of toothpaste) until the bowel is back in the abdominal cavity. This defect is associated with a high rate of mortality (25%), increased incidences of chromosomal abnormalities, and other severe malformations, such as cardiac (50%) and neural tube defects (25%). Another defect associated with the midgut involves its connection to the yolk sac via the vitelline duct. Normally, this duct degenerates, but sometimes a partial or complete connection is maintained resulting in a **diverticulum (Meckel's diverticulum),** a cyst, or a fistula at the umbilicus (**I–K**).

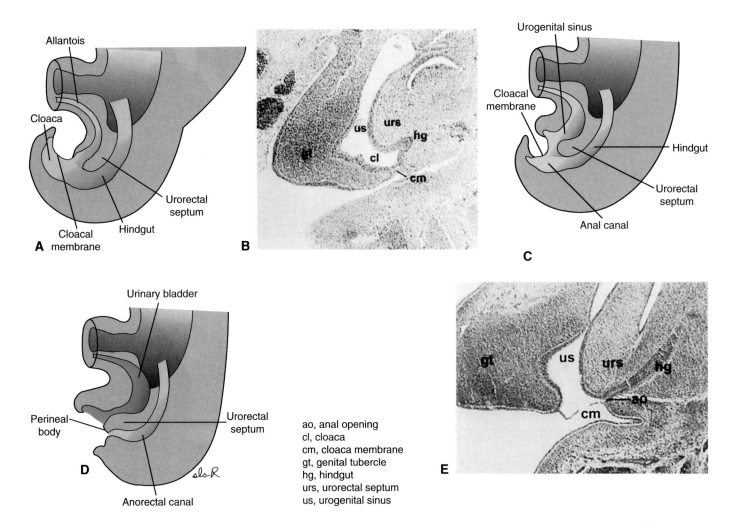

ao, anal opening
cl, cloaca
cm, cloaca membrane
gt, genital tubercle
hg, hindgut
urs, urorectal septum
us, urogenital sinus

FIGURE 6.8. The **hindgut** forms the left one third of the transverse colon, the descending colon, sigmoid colon, rectum, and the upper part of the anal canal. At 6 weeks gestation, the hindgut ends in a chamber called the **cloaca**, which is closed from the exterior by the **cloacal membrane** (**A** and **B**). The anterior portion of this chamber forms the **urogenital sinus**, while the posterior portion forms the **anorectal canal** (**C** and **D**). In the 6th week, these two regions become separated in part by a wedge of mesoderm called the **urorectal septum** that grows caudally between them and ends as the **perineal body** (**A–E**). At the end of the 7th week, the cloacal membrane degenerates (**E**), but at the same time proliferation of ectoderm at the end of the anus prevents the hindgut from opening to the exterior. In the 9th week, this ectodermal plug canalizes, creating the lower end of the anal canal. Thus, the upper end of the anal canal is derived from hindgut endoderm, whereas the lower end is derived from ectoderm. The junction between the two sections forms the **pectinate line**. Failure of canalization of the ectoderm results in **imperforate anus** (for discussion of other defects in this region, see Fig. 7.6). **B** and **E**: sections through human embryos at 6 weeks (**B**) and 7 weeks (**E**) gestation.

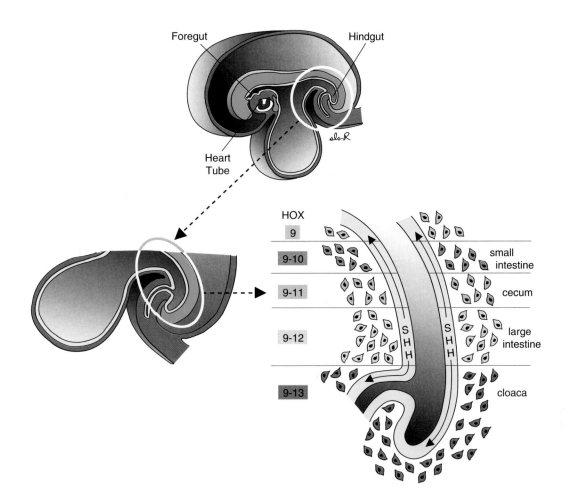

FIGURE 6.9. The molecular code responsible for differentiation of the various regions of the gut and its derivatives has been partially characterized. Development of all of these regions depends on reciprocal interactions between gut epithelium (endoderm) and the surrounding splanchnic mesoderm (epithelial–mesenchymal interactions). Mesoderm dictates the type of structure that forms, for example, lungs from the foregut and descending colon from the hindgut. Genetic instructions for this specification are carried by a *HOX* code, similar to the one that establishes specification along the cranial–caudal axis (see Fig. 3.9). Induction of the *HOX* code is elicited by *Sonic hedgehog (SHH)* expressed in gut endoderm along the entire length of the gut tube. In turn, SHH establishes a nested *HOX* gene expression pattern in the mesoderm that specifies the type of structure and differentiation that occurs. For example, the code for hindgut development is shown in the above figure. Similar codes are established in the midgut and foregut regions to pattern their differentiation. Variations in concentrations of SHH probably account for the specific pattern of organ formation along the gut tube.

CHAPTER 7

Urogenital System

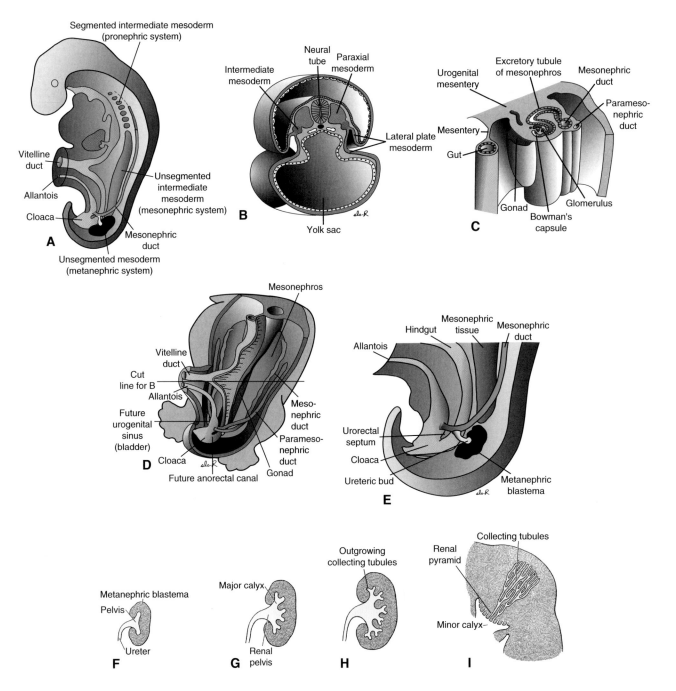

FIGURE 7.1. Development of the **urinary** and **genital** systems is intricately interwoven. Both of these systems are derived largely from a common ridge of **intermediate mesoderm** that lies along the posterior abdominal wall in a retroperitoneal position (**A** and **B**). The **functional unit** of the kidney is the **nephron** or **excretory unit**, which consists of a collection of capillaries called a **glomerulus** and a system of **excretory tubules** that filter and concentrate the urine (**C**; example of a nephron from the mesonephric kidney system). Nephrons connect to a system of **collecting ducts** to deliver urine for excretion (**C** and **D**). Three kidney systems develop sequentially. The first of these, the **pronephros**, is vestigial and never functions: it forms a few tubules in intermediate mesoderm in the cervical region in the 4th week and degenerates by the end of that week without ever having functioned (**A**). The second, the **mesonephros**, appears in thoracic and lumbar segments as the pronephros is degenerating and forms segmentally arranged nephrons (**B**) that empty into a collecting duct called the **mesonephric (Wolffian) duct**. This duct connects these primitive nephrons, a few of which may function for a short time, with the **urogenital sinus** (the future bladder; **C** and **D**). By the 6th week, thoracic segments of the mesonephros have degenerated, and the system is represented by an unsegmented ovoid mass of intermediate mesoderm that has the developing **gonad** (also derived from intermediate mesoderm) along its medial border (**D**). Together these structures comprise the **urogenital ridge**. Soon, however, most of the remaining parts of the mesonephric system degenerate, leaving only a few excretory tubules and the mesonephric duct in the male, and only vestigial remnants in the female (see Figs. 7.7 and 7.8). The **metanephros**, or definitive kidney, begins development at the end of the 5th week as the cranial-most parts of the mesonephros are degenerating (**A**). The metanephros has two components: (1) a collecting system that arises from the **ureteric bud**, an outgrowth from the caudal end of the mesonephric duct (**E**); and (2) the **metanephric mesoderm (metanephric blastema)**, a collection of intermediate mesoderm in the pelvic region (**E**). The ureteric bud grows out and contacts the metanephric mesoderm and then the two components interact to support each other's differentiation (see Fig. 7.2). Contact with the mesoderm causes the bud to expand and then to branch (**F–H**) into smaller and smaller divisions until 12 or more generations of tubules are created (**I**). The expanded portion forms the **renal pelvis**, while branches form the **major calyces, minor calyces,** and 1 to 3 million **collecting tubules** (**F–I**). Successive generations of collecting tubules converge on each of the minor calyces, creating the **renal pyramids** (**H** and **I**). Lengthening of the proximal end of each ureteric bud forms the **ureters**.

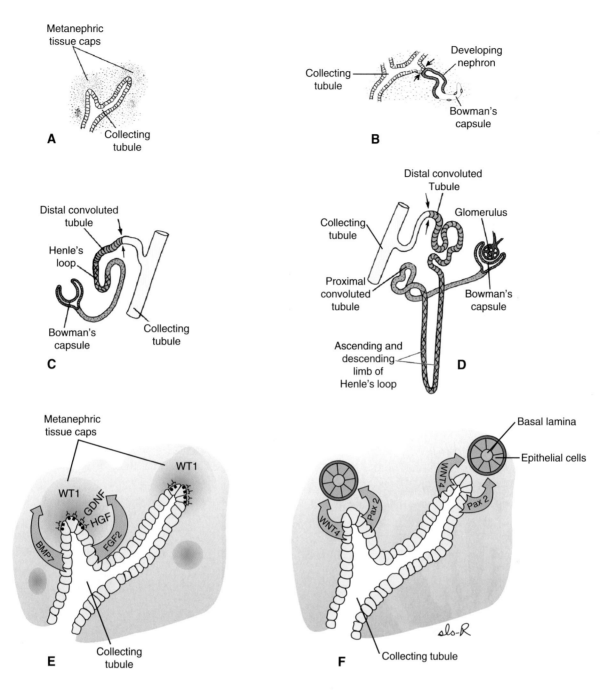

FIGURE 7.2. Meanwhile, mesoderm at the end of each **collecting tubule** forms a **metanephric tissue cap** that is induced by the tubules to form nephrons (**A** and **B**). Each tubule of a nephron develops a cup-like structure at its proximal end called **Bowman's capsule** (**B** and **C**), and this capsule fits around a tuft of capillaries called a **glomerulus** (**D**). Next, the tubules of the nephrons lengthen and differentiate into the **proximal convoluted tubule, loop of Henle**, and **distal convoluted tubule** (**D**). Distal convoluted tubules empty into collecting tubules (**D**), and these converge at the renal pyramids, where they empty into the minor calyces (Fig 7.1H). Molecular signals responsible for the crosstalk between the ureteric bud and metanephric mesoderm have been well characterized. Each of the metanephric tissue caps expresses *WT1*, a transcription factor and master gene for kidney development (**E**). *WT1* regulates production of glial-derived neurotrophic growth factor (GDNF) and hepatocyte growth factor (HGF, or scatter factor) by metanephric mesoderm, while tyrosine kinase receptors for these factors called RET (for GDNF) and MET (for HGF) are synthesized by epithelium of the ureteric bud (**E**). Thus, signaling pathways are established between these two tissue components by the secreted factors and their receptors. In turn, cells from the ureteric buds induce the metanephric mesoderm via fibroblast growth factor 2(FGF2) and bone morphogenetic protein 7 (BMP7; **E**). Both of these factors stimulate proliferation of metanephric mesoderm and maintain *WT1* expression. Conversion of metanephric mesoderm to epithelium for nephron tubule formation is signaled by the transcription factor PAX2 and the growth factor WNT4 (**F**). These signals cause changes in the extracellular matrix, such that fibronectin and collagen types I and II (mesenchymal type molecules) are replaced by laminin and type IV collagen (epithelial-type molecules for establishing a basal lamina; **F**). In addition, the cell adhesion molecules syndecan and E-cadherin are synthesized and used to assist in conversion of metanephric mesoderm from a mesenchymal to an epithelial cell type (**F**).

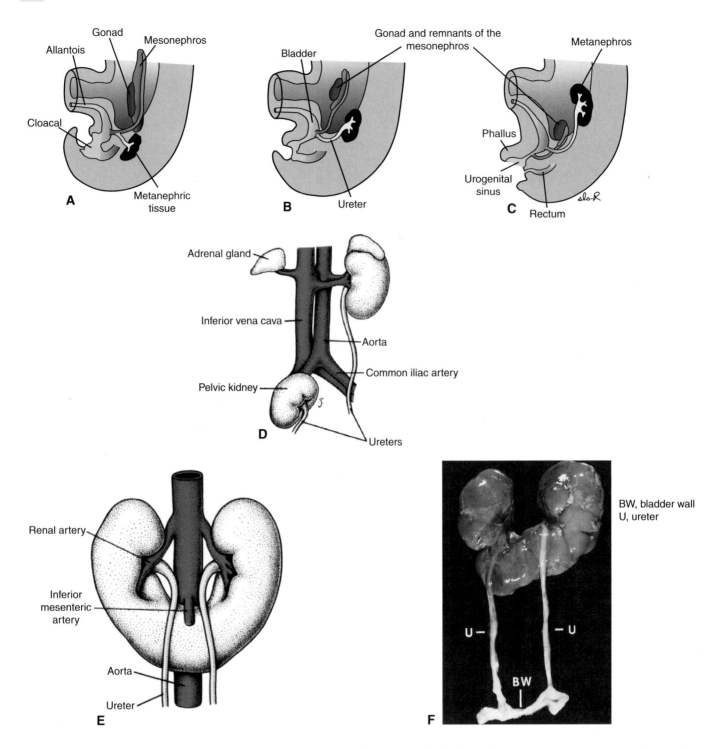

FIGURE 7.3.   Because metanephric mesoderm lies in the pelvic region, the kidneys have to move cranially to achieve their final position in the lower lumbar area. This "**ascent of the kidneys**" is caused more by differential growth—i.e., the kidneys stay in position, while the embryo lengthens—than by active movement of the kidneys themselves (**A–C**). Sometimes, a kidney or kidneys fails to "ascend" to the lumbar area, creating a **pelvic kidney (D)**. In other cases, the two areas of metanephric mesoderm located close together in the pelvic region, may fuse to form a **horseshoe kidney** (seen in 1 per 600 births; **E** and **F**). When this type of kidney starts to ascend it is trapped by the inferior mesenteric artery off of the aorta and stops at that position at the pelvic brim. Function of the kidneys begins in the 12th week. Amniotic fluid is swallowed by the fetus, absorbed from the gut into the bloodstream, filtered by the nephrons, and excreted, essentially unchanged, back into the amniotic fluid. Waste products that later will be excreted in the urine are removed by the placenta during fetal development.

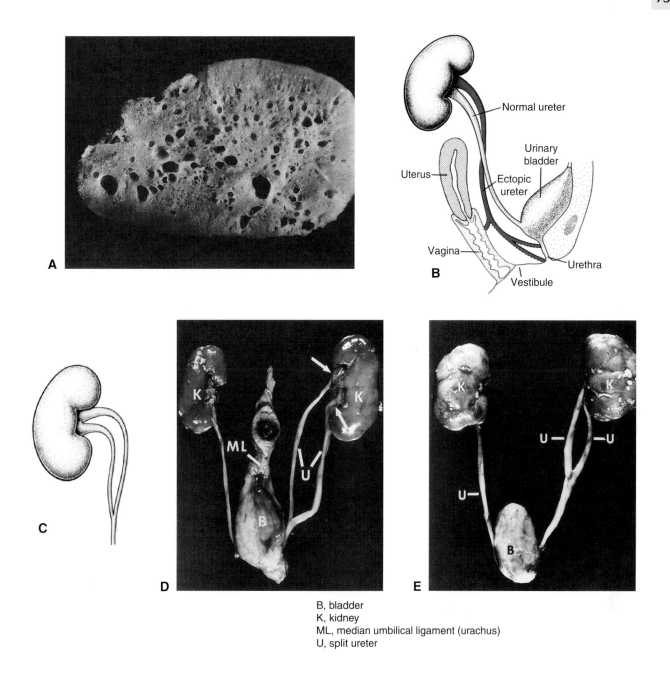

B, bladder
K, kidney
ML, median umbilical ligament (urachus)
U, split ureter

FIGURE 7.4.   A number of other birth defects involve the kidneys. In some cases (1 per 10,000 births), the ureteric bud fails to contact metanephric mesoderm, so that no kidney induction occurs, resulting in unilateral or bilateral **renal agenesis**. Bilateral cases are lethal and usually are associated with other major defects. Kidney tumors also may occur. Mutations in the *WT1* gene are responsible for **Wilms tumor**, a common cancer of early childhood. Wilms tumors usually form in the first 5 years of life, but may occur in the fetus. **Congenital polycystic kidneys** occur in an autosomal dominant or recessive form (**A**). The recessive form occurs in 1 per 5,000 births and is characterized as a progressive disorder in which multiple cysts form from collecting tubules, resulting in renal failure in infancy or early childhood. In the dominant form, which is more common (1 per 500 to 1,000 births) and less progressive, cysts form from all segments of the nephron and usually do not cause renal failure until adulthood. In rare cases, a ureter may open into the vagina or urethra (**ectopic ureters**) due to an abnormally low positioning of the ureteric bud on the mesonephric duct (**B**). In this situation, when the mesonephric duct is incorporated into the bladder (see Fig. 7.5), the ureter is too low and opens into one of the other neighboring structures. Duplications of the ureters may occur if there is a split in the ureteric bud (**C–E**; *arrows* in **D** indicate duplicated hilum). The resulting duplications may be partial or complete, depending on how early in development the split occurs.

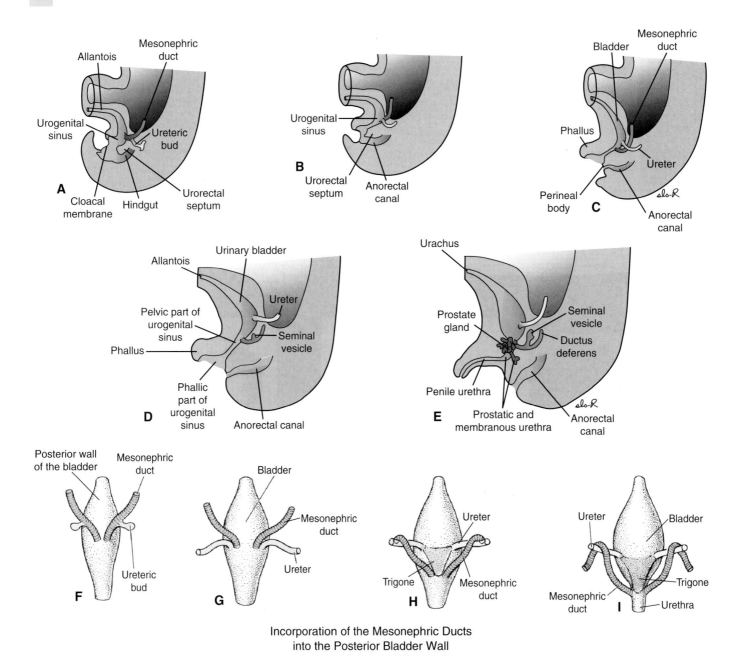

Incorporation of the Mesonephric Ducts
into the Posterior Bladder Wall

FIGURE 7.5. The **bladder** is derived from the anterior region of the cloaca called the **urogenital sinus** (**A**). Originally, the prospective bladder opens into this anterior part of the cloaca and the hindgut enters the posterior part (**A**). At the end of the 5th week, a wedge of mesoderm called the **urorectal septum** grows down and begins to separate the cloaca into the urogenital sinus and the **anal canal** (**A** and **B**). By 8 weeks, the separation is complete, and the tip of the urorectal septum forms the **perineal body** (**C**). At this time, three parts of the urogenital sinus can be identified. The **urinary bladder** is the upper and largest part, and it is continuous with the **allantois** (a vestigial organ that serves a respiratory function in avian embryos), which passes out the umbilicus. Later, the allantois degenerates to a fibrous cord called the **urachus**, which forms the median umbilical ligament (**D** and **E**). The pelvic portion forms the **prostatic** and **membranous urethra** in the male (**D** and **E**), and the **phallic part** forms the **penile urethra** in the male (**D** and **E**). During expansion of the urogenital sinus, the **mesonephric ducts** are absorbed into the wall of the urinary bladder. Consequently, the **ureters**, which originally arose from the mesonephric ducts as the ureteric buds, come to open directly into the bladder (**A–C** and **F–I**). Caudally, the mesonephric ducts move closer together to enter the prostatic portion of the urethra, where they form the **ejaculatory ducts** in the male (**E**). In females, the mesonephric ducts degenerate, leaving only a few vestigial remnants (see Fig. 7.8). Incorporation of the mesonephric ducts into the bladder creates a triangular region on this structure's posterior wall called the **trigone** (**H** and **I**). Because the mesonephric ducts are mesodermal in origin (intermediate mesoderm), whereas the cloaca is endodermal (essentially, the end of the hindgut), the bladder has a dual origin. At the end of the 3rd month, cells in the urethral epithelium, just distal to the neck of the bladder, differentiate into the **prostate gland** (**E**). In females, this portion of the urethra forms the **urethral** and **paraurethral glands**. Finally, in males, **seminal vesicles** form as outgrowths from the mesonephric ducts (**E**).

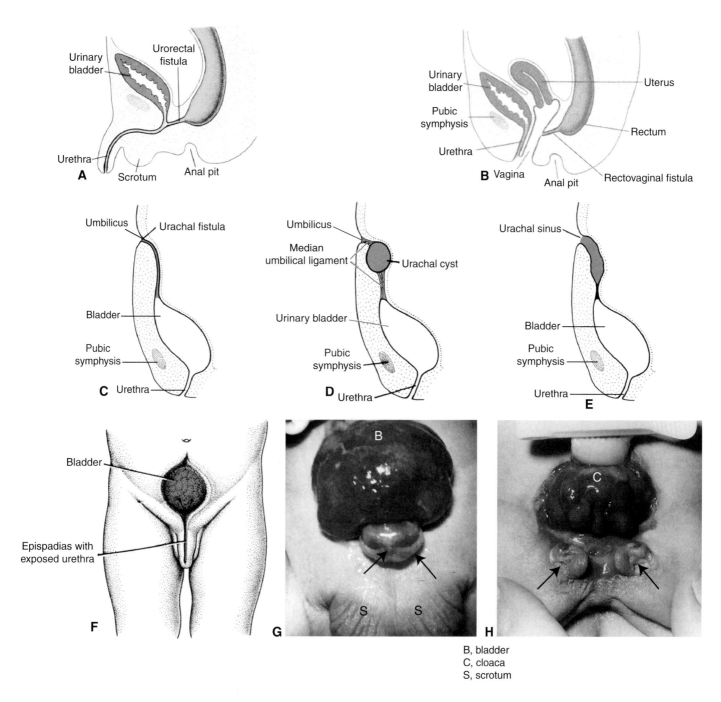

B, bladder
C, cloaca
S, scrotum

FIGURE 7.6. Birth defects in the cloacal region include **urorectal** and **rectovaginal fistulas** that are due to incomplete separation of the anal canal from the urogenital sinus (1 per 5,000 births). This lack of separation may be due to a failure of the urorectal septum to grow downward sufficiently (Fig. 7.5A–C) or to the fact that the original cloacal chamber was too small, leaving no room for formation of the anal canal. In either case, the opening of the hindgut is shifted anteriorly toward the urogenital sinus. As a result, the hindgut empties directly into the urethra in the male, forming a urorectal fistula (**A**), or into the vagina in females, forming a rectovaginal fistula (**B**). Other defects involve a failure of the allantois to degenerate. This failure results in formation of urachal fistulas (**C**), cysts (**D**), and sinuses (**E**). In some cases, body folding is not completed in the pelvic region because the two lateral folds and the tail fold do not come together. Such an occurrence causes a ventral body wall defect in which either the bladder (**bladder extrophy**; F and **G**; *arrows* in **G** indicate a penis with epispadias) or the cloaca (**cloacal extrophy**; **H**; *arrows* in **H** indicate genital swellings) is exposed. Bladder extrophy is less common (1 per 200,000 births) and less severe, although it is always accompanied by epispadius, a condition in which there is an opening along the dorsum of the penis such that the urethra is exposed (**F** and **G**). In contrast, cloacal extrophy occurs more often (1 per 30,000 births), is more severe, and usually is accompanied by spinal defects and omphalocele.

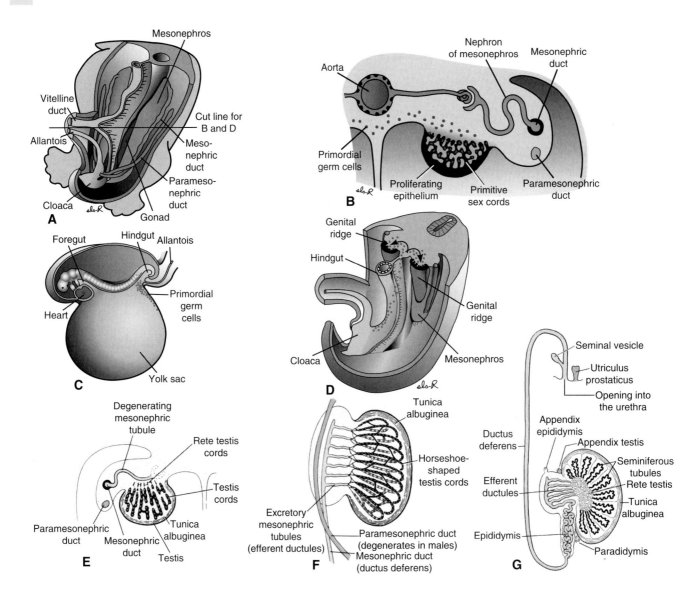

FIGURE 7.7. The fate of genital system development depends on whether or not a **Y chromosome** is present. This chromosome contains the *SRY* **(sex-determining region on Y) gene**, a transcription factor that regulates male development. The *SRY* gene is the **testis determining factor**. Under its influence male development occurs, whereas in its absence, female development takes place. In either case, however, early stages of gonad and external genitalia development are the same, for both sexes. **Gonads** first appear as gonadal ridges formed in intermediate mesoderm along the medial border of the mesonephric system at the end of the 4th week (**A** and **B**). Together these structures form the **urogenital ridge**. Soon after the gonadal ridges appear, epithelial cells covering the ridge proliferate and penetrate the underlying mesoderm to form **primitive sex cords** (**B**). At about the same time, **primordial germ cells** (future eggs or sperm) differentiate in the wall of the yolk sac near the allantois (**C**) and begin to migrate along this structure and then the dorsal mesentery of the hindgut toward the gonadal ridges (**D**). Here, they arrive in the 5th week (**D**), penetrate the ridges in the 6th week, and become surrounded by epithelial cells of the primitive sex cords (**B**). If the embryo is male, these sex cords continue to proliferate toward the center (medulla) of the testis to form the **testis** or **medullary cords** (**E**). At their proximal ends, they form tiny tubules called, collectively, the **rete testis**, and they become separated from the surface by a tough fibrous tissue that covers the testis, the **tunica albuginea** (**E**). In the 4th month, the cords become horseshoe-shaped, maintain their connection to the rete testis, and continue to house the primordial germ cells (**F**). In addition, some of the epithelial cells in the cords differentiate into **Sertoli cells**, which are important for germ cell differentiation into sperm. Even before the appearance of Sertoli cells, some mesoderm cells lying between the cords differentiate into **interstitial cells (of Leydig)**, and these cells begin **testosterone** production by the 8th week. Testis cords remain solid until puberty, when a lumen forms and they differentiate into **seminiferous tubules** where sperm are produced (**G**). These tubules maintain their connections with the rete testis, which, in turn, connect to the **efferent ductules**. Efferent ductules are derived from some of the nephric tubules of the mesonephric system that lie in close proximity to the testis, and these empty into the original mesonephric duct, which now becomes the **ductus deferens** for sperm transport (**G**). The remaining mesonephric tubules and the cranial end of the duct degenerate, leaving only remnants called the paradidymis and appendix epididymis, respectively (**G**). Later, part of the mesonephric duct distal to the efferent ductules becomes highly convoluted and forms the **epididymis**, where sperm are stored prior to ejaculation (**G**).

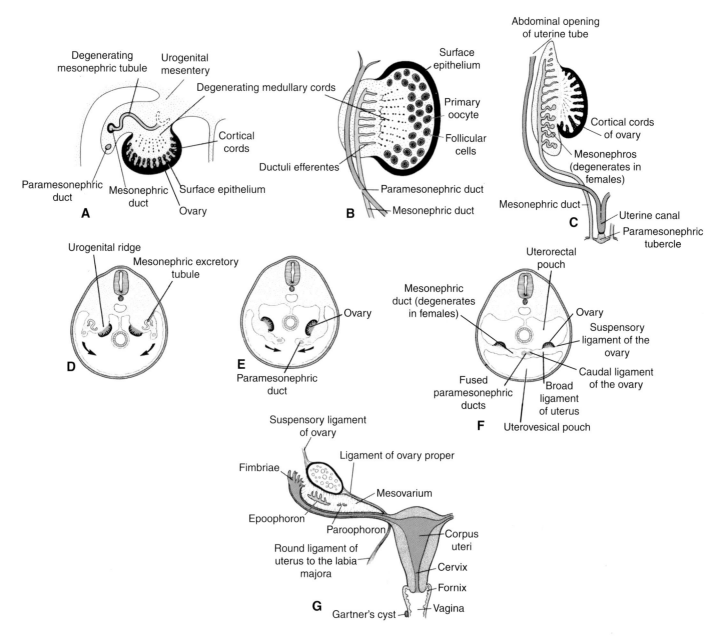

FIGURE 7.8. In the **ovary**, primitive sex cords penetrate to the medulla but then degenerate (**A**). Then, in the 7th week, the surface epithelium of the ovary forms a second set of cords, called the **cortical cords**, that remain close to the surface in the cortex (**A**). In the 4th month, these cords split into isolated clusters, each surrounding one or more **germ cells**. Subsequently, germ cells develop into **oogonia (eggs)**, and the surrounding epithelial cells differentiate into **follicular cells** (**B**). Another difference in females is that the **mesonephric system** degenerates (except for a few vestigial remnants called the epoophoron, paroophoron, and Gartner's cyst; see **G**), while a second duct system develops. These second ducts are called the **paramesonephric ducts (müllerian ducts)** because they develop beside (para) the mesonephric ducts (**B** and **C**). (A paramesonephric system also develops in males, but degenerates, leaving only vestigial remnants called the prostatic utricle and appendix testis; see Fig. 7.7G). The paramesonephric ducts open to the peritoneal cavity cranially and contact the urogenital sinus caudally in close proximity to each other (**A** and **C**). Then, due to growth of the urogenital ridges that shifts the position of the ovary into the abdominal cavity (but still retroperitoneal; **D–F**), the lower ends of the ducts fuse to form the **uterus** and upper portion of the **vagina** (**C–G**). These ridges are covered by a layer of peritoneum as they grow toward the midline, and this layer is carried with the ridges to fuse and form a broad sheet of mesentery, the **broad ligament of the uterus**, across the abdominal cavity (**F**). This sheet effectively divides the pelvis into the **uterorectal pouch** posteriorly and the **uterovesical (bladder) pouch** anteriorly (**F**). **Suspensory** and **caudal ovarian ligaments** condense from urogenital ridge mesoderm to form fibrous cords to support the ovary (**F**). Later, when the uterus grows larger, the caudal ligament attaches to its wall to form the **proper ovarian ligament** proximally and the **round ligament of the uterus** caudally (**G**). Cranially, the paramesonephric ducts lengthen to form the **uterine tubes (fallopian tubes)** with their openings and surrounding **fimbriae** next to the ovary (**G**). The ovary and uterine tubes are covered by peritoneum (broad ligament), but the tubes open into the peritoneal cavity. Therefore, during ovulation, eggs rupture through the peritoneal covering of the ovary to enter the peritoneal cavity, where they are swept into the uterine tubes by the fimbriae.

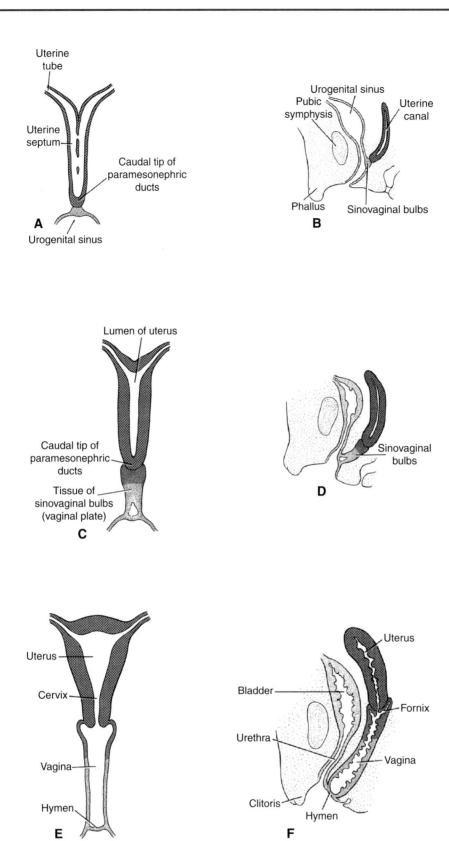

FIGURE 7.9. As mentioned earlier, fusion of the lower portion of the paramesonephric ducts forms the uterus and upper part of the vagina. The lower part of the vagina is derived from the posterior wall of the urogenital sinus (**A** and **B**). The anterior portion of the urogenital sinus forms the bladder and urethra (see Fig. 7.5). Contact of the urogenital sinus by the paramesonephric ducts induces formation of the **sinovaginal bulbs** (**C** and **D**). These bulbs are a collection of endoderm cells from the wall of the urogenital sinus that proliferate to form a solid column of tissue in the 3rd month (**C** and **D**). In the 5th month, this tissue canalizes to form the lower part of the vagina (**E** and **F**). During canalization, the hymen forms as a thin membrane with a centrally located opening (**E** and **F**).

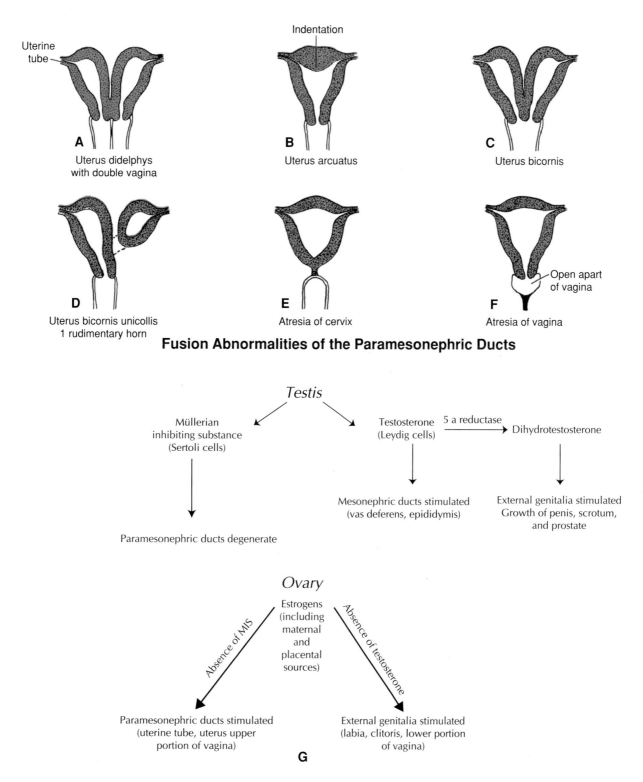

Fusion Abnormalities of the Paramesonephric Ducts

FIGURE 7.10. Fusion abnormalities of the paramesonephric ducts (**A–F**) may cause birth defects involving the uterus or vagina (or both) that can lead to problems with fertility or menstruation. Development of the reproductive duct system and differentiation of the external genitalia are controlled by hormones and hormone-like substances (**G**). In males, **interstitial cells of Leydig** produce **testosterone**, which stimulates differentiation of the mesonephric system. In addition, Sertoli cells in the seminiferous tubules of the testis produce **müllerian-inhibiting substance** (**MIS**; also called **antimüllerian hormone**), which causes regression of the **paramesonephric (müllerian) duct**. Testosterone also directs development of the male external genitalia, but it is first converted to **dihydrotestosterone**. In females, the absence of testosterone causes regression of the mesonephric ducts, while the absence of MIS, plus the presence of **estrogen**, stimulates development of the **paramesonephric (müllerian) system**. Estrogens also assist in directing differentiation of the external genitalia.

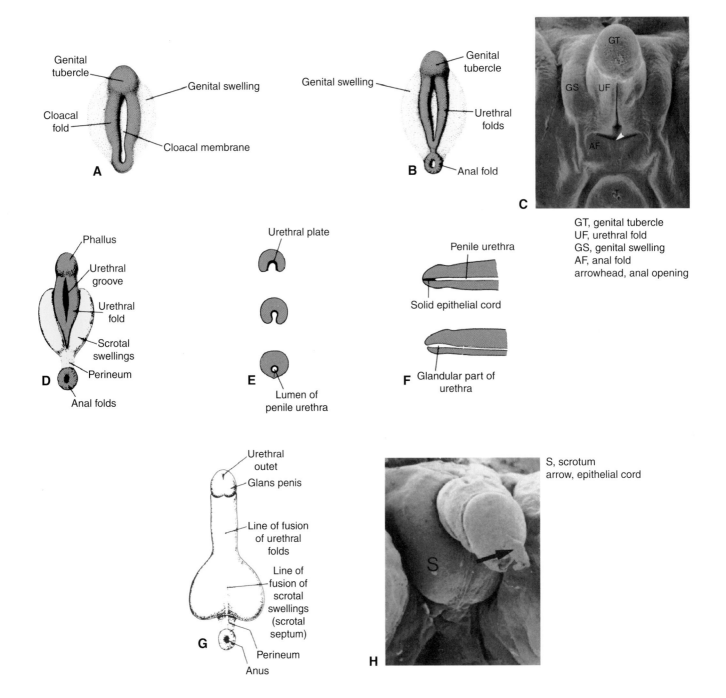

FIGURE 7.11. Like the gonads, the **external genitalia** in both sexes begin their differentiation along identical paths. Thus, at 4 weeks, there is a proliferation of mesoderm around the **cloacal membrane** that forms the **cloacal folds (A)**. Cranially, these folds unite to form the **genital tubercle (A)**. By 6 weeks, as the cloaca is separated into the anal canal and urogenital sinus and the cloacal membrane breaks down (see Fig. 7.5), the cloacal folds differentiate into the anal and urethral folds surrounding the openings into these two structures (**B** and **C**). In addition, a second set of elevations, called the genital swellings, forms lateral to the urethral folds (**B** and **C**). At this stage, called the **indifferent stage**, it is impossible to distinguish males from females by these landmarks. However, over the next several weeks, distinguishing changes occur. In males, under the influence of **dihydrotestosterone**, the genital tubercle, which is now called the **phallus**, lengthens to form the **penis**, and as it does so, it pulls the **urethral folds** with it (**D**). These folds then fuse along the ventral aspect of the penis to create the **penile urethra (D–F)**. However, this canal does not extend all the way to the tip of the penis. This portion of the urethra forms by a proliferation of ectodermal cells at the tip that create a solid epithelial cord in this region (**F**). Later, the cord canalizes to form the **external urethral meatus** and most of the glandular portion of the urethra (**F** and **G**). Meanwhile, the **genital swellings** enlarge to become the **scrotal swellings (D)**. These continue to enlarge until they fuse in the midline ventral to the penis to form the **scrotum**.

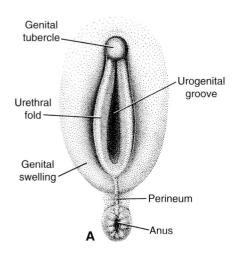

A

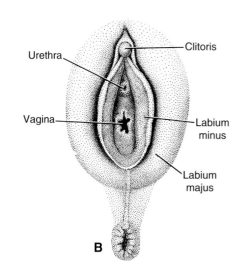

B

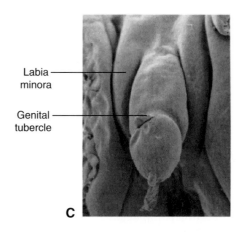

C

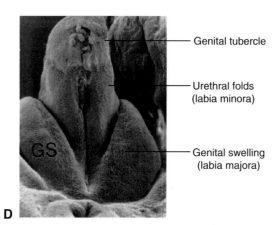

D

FIGURE 7.12. In females, the **genital tubercle** does not lengthen as extensively and forms the **clitoris**; while the **urethral folds** remain unfused and form the **labia minora** that flank the openings for the **urethra** and **vagina** (**A** and **B**). This area, bordered by the labia minora, is called the **vestibule**. The **genital swellings** enlarge, but also fail to fuse, thereby forming the **labia majora** (**A** and **B**). At early stages (up to 14 weeks), development of this region in females (**C** and **D**; both are of female genitalia) appears similar to that of males. It is so similar, in fact, that it is not possible to make a reliable determination of the baby's sex using ultrasound at this time.

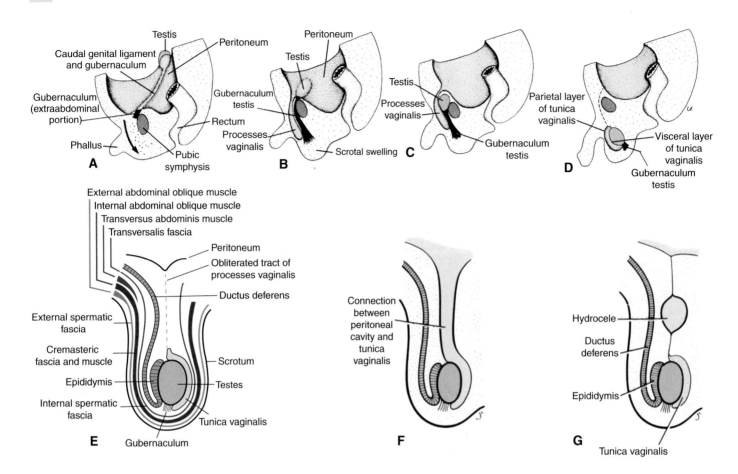

FIGURE 7.13. Both the **testes** and the **ovaries** develop retroperitoneally as part of the urogenital ridge along the posterior abdominal wall (see Fig. 7.1). Both also descend caudally, with the testes moving all the way to the scrotum and the ovaries (see Fig. 7.8). only a short distance. As they develop, the **caudal genital ligament**, composed of fibrous tissue derived from urogenital ridge mesoderm, forms and attaches from their caudal poles to the genital swellings (scrotum and labia majora; **A**). When the uterus forms, the caudal ligament is interrupted in its course by growth of the uterus and becomes attached to the uterine wall. The part of the ligament from the ovary to this wall forms the **proper ligament of the ovary**, while the part extending from the wall to the labia majora forms the **round ligament of the uterus** (Fig. 7.8F and G). In addition, a **cranial ovarian ligament**, the **suspensory ligament**, forms from urogenital ridge mesoderm to hold the ovary in place at this pole (Fig. 7.8F and G). In males, the caudal genital ligament becomes surrounded by a band of mesenchyme tissue called the **gubernaculum testis** (**A**). Initially, this tissue band terminates in the **inguinal region**, but later it grows down to the floor of the **scrotum** (**B**). The gubernaculum is largely responsible for pulling the testes into the scrotum. Thus, outgrowth of the gubernaculum from the inguinal region to the scrotum pulls the testes to the inguinal area (**B**); then, as organ growth occurs and intra-abdominal pressure increases, the testes are pushed into and through the inguinal canal (**C**). Finally, regression (shortening) of the gubernaculum from the scrotum to the inguinal canal pulls the testes into the scrotal sac (**D**). The testes reach the inguinal region by 12 weeks, pass through the inguinal canal by 28 weeks, and reach the scrotum by 33 weeks. To pass from their intra-abdominal position of origin to the scrotum, the testes must migrate through the abdominal wall via the **inguinal canal**. They are preceded in this maneuver by an outpocketing of peritoneum called the **processes vaginalis** (**B** and **C**). As this process migrates through the wall, it is accompanied by abdominal wall muscle and fascial layers and forms the inguinal canal. The testes migrate along this same path and become covered by these muscle and fascial layers as well. In addition, once the testes reach the scrotum, they are partially enveloped by the processes vaginalis that now forms the **tunica vaginalis** with a visceral layer (next to the testis) and a parietal layer (**C** and **D**). Coverings of the testes that are derived from constituents of the abdominal wall include the transversalis fascia, which forms the **internal spermatic fascia**; the internal abdominal oblique muscle, which gives rise to the **cremasteric fascia and muscle**; and the external abdominal oblique muscle, which forms the **external spermatic fascia** (**E**). The other muscle layer of the abdominal wall is the transversus abdominis muscle, but it does not contribute a layer because it arches over the internal ring of the inguinal canal and, thus, does not cover the path of migration. Normally, the connection between the processes vaginalis and the peritoneal cavity (**B** and **C**) is obliterated. If it is not, then intestinal loops may descend into or through the inguinal canal to the scrotum, forming a **congenital inguinal (indirect) hernia** (**F**). Occasionally this connection is only partially closed, leaving a cyst that may secrete fluid, creating a hydrocele of the spermatic cord or testis (**G**). In 97 % of male newborns, the testes are present in the scrotum at birth; in most others their descent will be completed by the age of 3 months. In some boys (<1 %), however, one or both testes fail to descend, a condition called **cryptorchidism**.

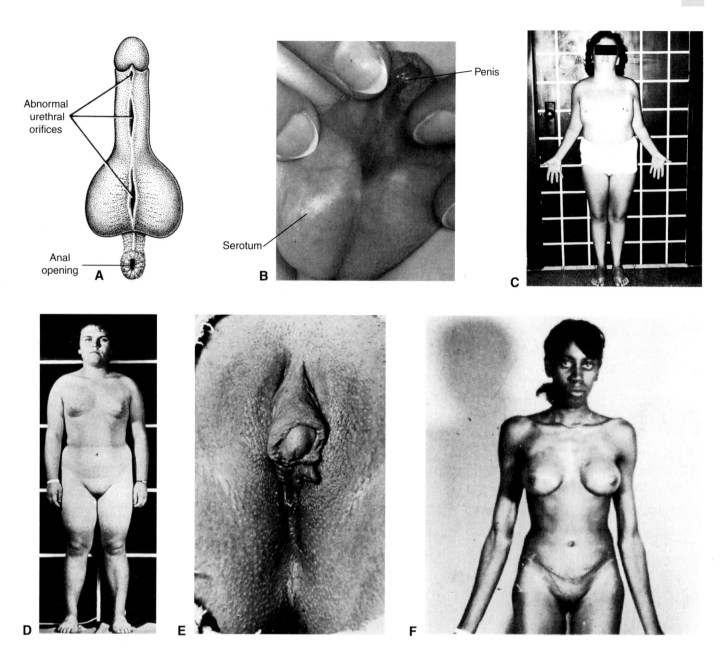

FIGURE 7.14. Many types of birth defects involve the genital system and may be due to genetic anomalies or teratogens. **Hypospadias** is a condition in which the urethral folds fail to fuse along the ventral aspect of the penis. The defect may occur anywhere along the shaft or root of the penis (**A** and **B**). Evidence suggests that the incidence of this defect is increasing, and some blame an increase in environmental estrogen-like compounds (**endocrine disruptors**). In another condition called **gonadal dysgenesis**, the ovaries are rudimentary structures and oocytes are absent. Individuals are phenotypically female, but may have a variety of chromosomal complements. In one such example, called XY female gonadal dysgenesis (Swyer syndrome), the condition is due to mutations or deletions in the *SRY* gene. In another example, patients with Turner syndrome have gonadal dysgenesis with a 45,X karyotype. The syndrome usually is associated with other defects, including shield-like chest, inverted nipples, short stature, webbed neck, and cardiac and renal anomalies (**C**). In cases of **pseudohermaphroditism**, individuals are unambiguous with respect to their gonadal sex and possess either testes or ovaries, but have ambiguous external genitalia. **Female pseudohermaphrodism** most often is caused by **congenital adrenal gland hyperplasia (adrenogenital syndrome)** in which the adrenal glands, due to a biochemical abnormality, produce androgen-like compounds. Patients have a 46,XX complement of chromosomes and ovaries, but have masculinization of the external genitalia, including clitoral hypertrophy and partial fusion of the labia majora (**D** and **E**). Male pseudohermaphrodites have a 46,XY chromosome complement, but fail to produce sufficient androgenic hormones and müllerian inhibiting substance (MIS). Thus, their internal and external sex characteristics vary depending on the concentrations of hormones that are produced. In another example of **male pseudohermaphrodism**, called **androgen insensitivity syndrome (testicular feminization)**, patients have a normal 46,XY karyotype, but have the external appearance of females (**F**). The problem is due to a lack of androgen (dihydrotestosterone) receptors or receptor responses in tissues that form the external genitalia.

CHAPTER 8

Craniofacial Development

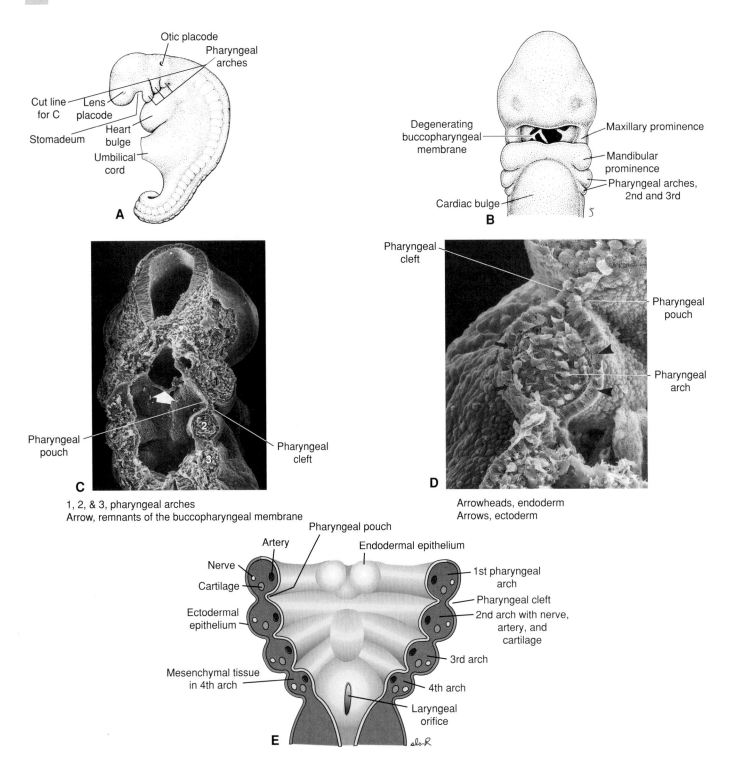

FIGURE 8.1. Cells and tissues for craniofacial development begin forming during early stages of gastrulation through the time of neural tube closure. Thus, by 4 weeks, when cranial neural folds have closed, the head region is distinguished by the presence of three brain vesicles; lens and otic placodes for eye and ear development; a primitive oral cavity, called the stomadeum, that is separated from the pharynx by the buccopharyngeal membrane; and three pairs of **pharyngeal arches** (**A** and **B**). Ultimately, five well-developed pairs of these pharyngeal arches, I, II, III, IV, and VI (the 5th pair is vestigial) form in a cranial-to-caudal sequence. Each arch consists of a core of mesenchyme, composed of mesoderm and neural crest cells, covered externally by ectoderm (*arrows* in **D**) and internally by endoderm (**C**; *arrowheads* in **D**). Each arch also has its own **aortic arch vessel** (see Fig. 5.10) and its own **cranial nerve** (**E**; Table 8.1). Externally, arches are separated by indentations called **pharyngeal clefts**; internally, they are separated by indentations called **pharyngeal pouches** (**D** and **E**). Thus, the arches appear as separate columns, but there are no openings between them because the clefts and pouches are covered by ectoderm and endoderm, respectively (**C–E**). (In fish, the arches would form gills and the intervening tissue would degenerate to create openings for water to pass through.) Each of the arches in the first pair forms two subdivisions, the **maxillary prominence** and the **mandibular process** (**A** and **B**, see also Fig.8.6C). (continued)

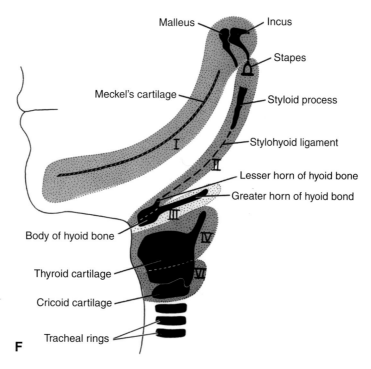

F

Table 8.1. **Derivatives of the Pharyngeal Arches and Their Innervation**

Pharyngeal Arch	Nerve	Muscles	Skeleton
1 mandibular (maxillary and mandibular processes)	V. Trigeminal: maxillary and mandibular divisions	Mastication (temporal; masseter; medial, lateral pterygoids); mylohyoid; anterior belly of digastric; tensor palatine, tensor tympani	Premaxilla, maxilla, zygomatic bone, part of temporal bone, Meckel's cartilage, mandible malleus, incus, anterior ligament of malleus, sphenomandibular ligament
2 hyoid	VII. Facial	Facial expression (buccinator; auricularis; frontalis; platysma; orbicularis oris; orbicularis oculi); posterior belly of digastric; stylohyoid; stapedius	Stapes; styloid process; stylohyoid ligament; lesser horn and upper portion of body of hyoid bone
3	IX. Glossopharyngeal	Stylopharyngeus	Greater horn and lower portion of body of hyoid bone
4–6	X. Vagus Superior laryngeal branch (nerve to 4th arch) Recurrent laryngeal branch (nerve to 6th arch)	Cricothyroid; levator palatine; constrictors of pharynx Intrinsic muscles of larynx	Laryngeal cartilages (thyroid, cricoid, arytenoid, corniculate, cuneiform)

FIGURE 8.1. (*Continued*) The arches themselves each form specific skeletal (derived from neural crest cells; **F**) and muscular (derived from paraxial mesoderm) components of the face (Table 8.1). The cranial nerve in each specific arch supplies the muscles that differentiate from that arch (Table 8.1).

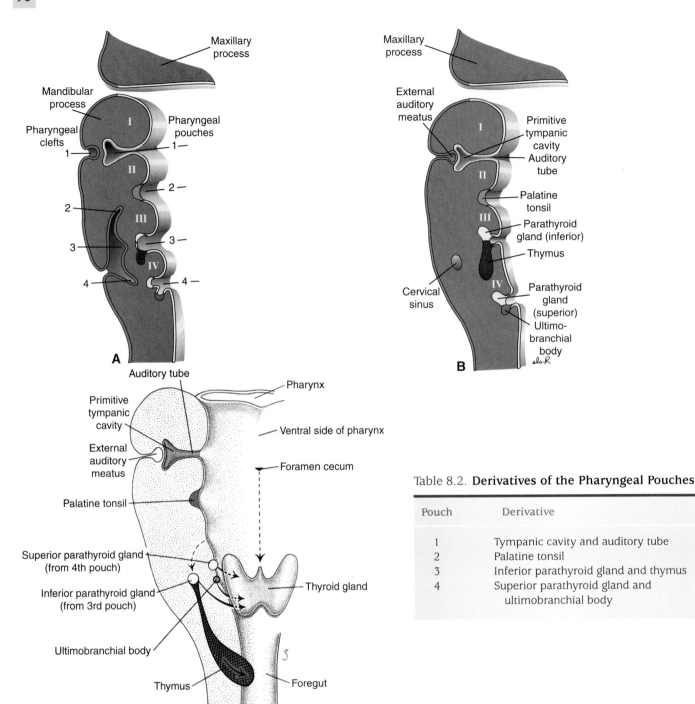

Table 8.2. **Derivatives of the Pharyngeal Pouches**

Pouch	Derivative
1	Tympanic cavity and auditory tube
2	Palatine tonsil
3	Inferior parathyroid gland and thymus
4	Superior parathyroid gland and ultimobranchial body

FIGURE 8.2.   The **1st pharyngeal cleft** lengthens medially to form the **external auditory meatus**, while the ectoderm–endoderm membrane between the 1st cleft and 1st pouch becomes the **tympanic membrane (eardrum; A and B;** see Fig. 10.6). The remainder of the clefts are overgrown by tissue of the second arch and disappear (**A and B**). The **1st pouch** expands laterally to form the **tubotympanic recess.** Distally, this recess expands to form the **middle ear cavity,** which is separated from the 1st cleft by the tympanic membrane (**A and B**). Proximally it lengthens and narrows to form the **auditory (eustachian) tube (A and B).** Endoderm of the remaining pouches proliferates and interacts with arch mesenchyme to form glands (**A–C**; Table 8.2). This interaction is similar to what occurs in the development of gut derivatives, such that endoderm forms the **glandular epithelium (parenchyma),** and mesenchyme (derived from neural crest cells) forms the **connective tissue stroma.** Due to migration of some of this glandular tissue, rearrangements from the expected pattern occur. For example, the thymus forms from the caudal part of the 3rd pouch and migrates to the thorax (**B and C**). As it does so, parathyroid tissue, that also develops from this pouch, migrates with the thymic tissue until it lies caudal to parathyroid-forming tissue originating from the 4th pouch. In this manner, parathyroids from the 3rd pouch form the inferior parathyroid glands, while those from the 4th pouch form the superior parathyroid glands (**C**). Migration of glandular tissue also explains the origin of ectopic parathyroid or thymic tissue that may occur in cervical or thoracic regions.

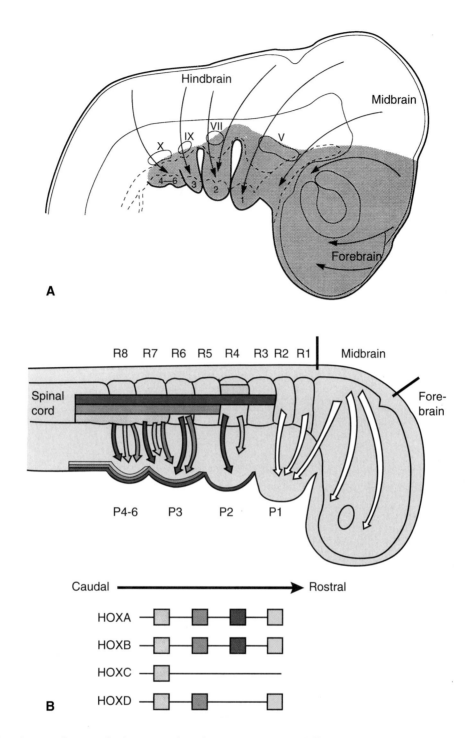

FIGURE 8.3. Molecular regulation of **pharyngeal arch** patterning and differentiation is dependent on migrating **neural crest cells** that carry a code of ***HOX* gene expression** similar to the one that establishes the body axis (Fig. 3.9B). These crest cells originate in the neural folds in the prospective hindbrain and midbrain regions and migrate to the pharyngeal arches (**A**; *arrows*). The hindbrain itself is segmented into eight regions called **rhombomeres** (R1–R8) that are patterned by an overlapping *HOX* code (**B**). Crest cells migrate from these rhombomeres to the pharyngeal arches (P1-P4-6) carrying the same code with them (**B**). Maintenance of the expression of this code depends on the interaction between crest cells and arch mesoderm. This interaction and expression of the code then determines the specificity of structures derived from each arch.

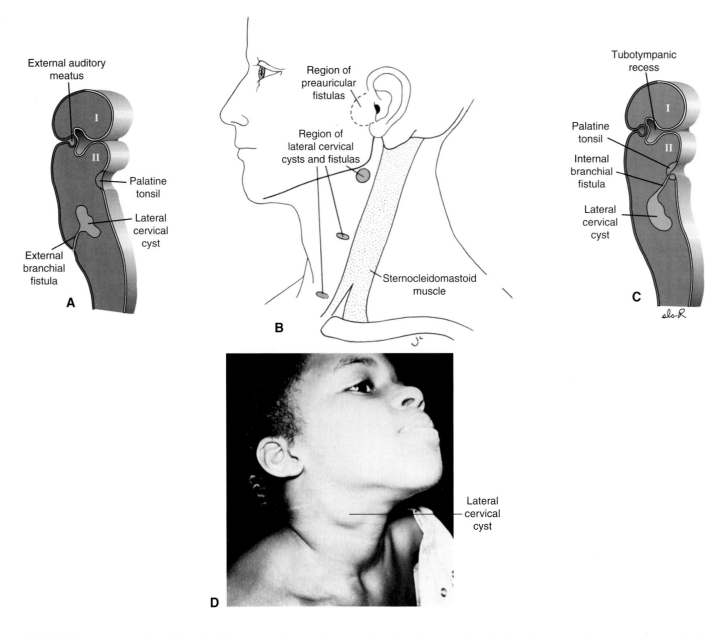

FIGURE 8.4. A number of birth defects are due to abnormalities in pharyngeal arch development. For example, cervical cysts and fistulas may arise along the anterior border of the sternocleidomastoid muscle due to improper closure of the pharyngeal clefts by 2nd arch overgrowth (**A–C**). Cysts are more common than fistulas (**D**).

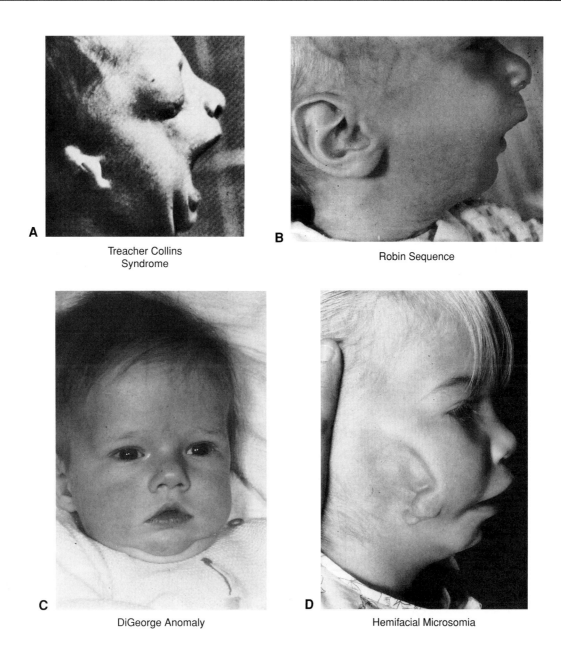

A   Treacher Collins Syndrome

B   Robin Sequence

C   DiGeorge Anomaly

D   Hemifacial Microsomia

FIGURE 8.5. Severe facial defects also may arise because of abnormal neural crest cell migration or differentiation, and they often are accompanied by cardiac defects, because crest cells also participate in heart development (see Fig. 5.7). Examples of these defects include Treacher-Collins syndrome, Robin sequence, DiGeorge syndrome, and hemifacial microsomia. **Treacher-Collins syndrome** (mandibulofacial dysostosis; **A**) is characterized by mandibular and malar hypoplasia due to underdevelopment of the mandible and zygomatic (1st arch) bones, eyelid colobomas, and malformed ears. It usually is inherited as an autosomal dominant trait. The **Robin sequence** (**B**) includes the triad of micrognathia (small mandible), glossoptosis (posteriorly placed tongue), and cleft palate. It may be caused by genetic or environmental factors, but the primary alteration is poor mandibular development. Because the mandible is small, the tongue lies more posteriorly and, by its physical presence, prevents fusion of the palatal shelves (see Fig. 8.7); **DiGeorge syndrome** (**C**) usually is due to a deletion on chromosome 22 and includes cardiac defects, abnormal facies, thymic hypoplasia, cleft palate, and hypocalcemia. Patients with severe DiGeorge syndrome have immunologic deficiencies (thymus), hypocalcemia (parathyroids and ultimobranchial body), and a poor prognosis. **Hemifacial microsomia** (e.g., **oculoauriculovertebral syndrome**, **Goldenhar syndrome**; **D**) involves a number of abnormalities, including small maxillary, temporal, or zygomatic bones; absent (anotia) or small (microtia) ears; eye anomalies (tumors and dermoids); and vertebral defects (e.g., fused or hemivertebrae, spina bifida). Facial asymmetry is present in 65% of these cases. All of these syndromes may be genetic or teratogen-induced. Teratogens that produce these malformations include retinoids, alcohol, and maternal diabetes.

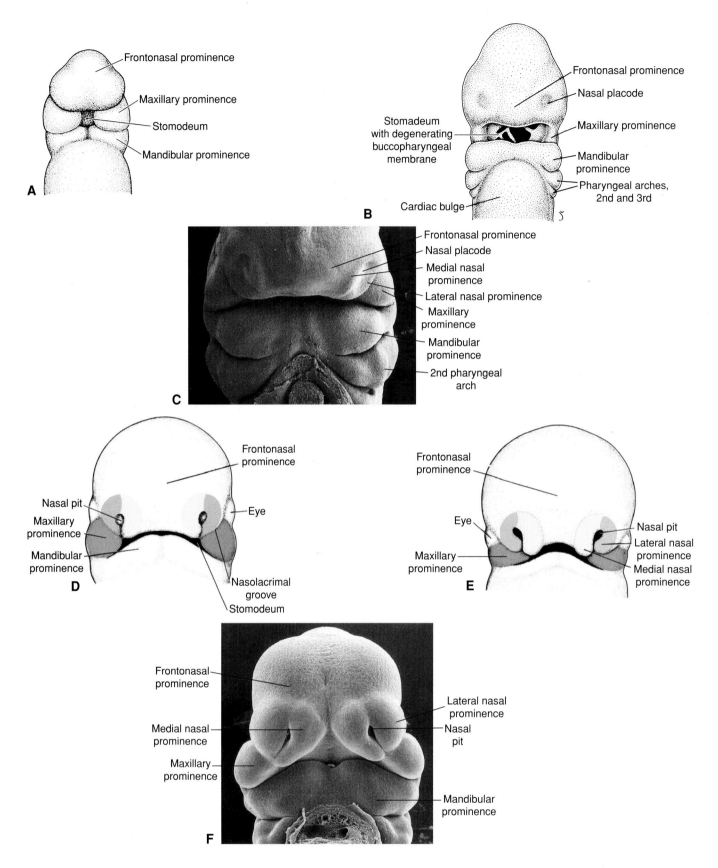

FIGURE 8.6. By the end of the 4th week, **facial prominences** are present. These include the paired **maxillary** and **mandibular prominences**, derived from the 1st arch, and the **frontonasal prominence** in the midline (**A**). At 4 1/2 weeks, **nasal (olfactory) placodes** (regions of thickened ectoderm) develop on both sides of the frontonasal prominence (**B** and **C**). These placodes invaginate to form the **nasal pits**, while tissue around them grows, creating two additional prominences, the **medial** and **lateral nasal prominences** (**C** and **D**). During the next 2 weeks, all of these prominences contribute to development of the face. The maxillary prominences increase in size and grow medially, pushing the medial nasal prominences closer together in the midline (**D–F**). (continued)

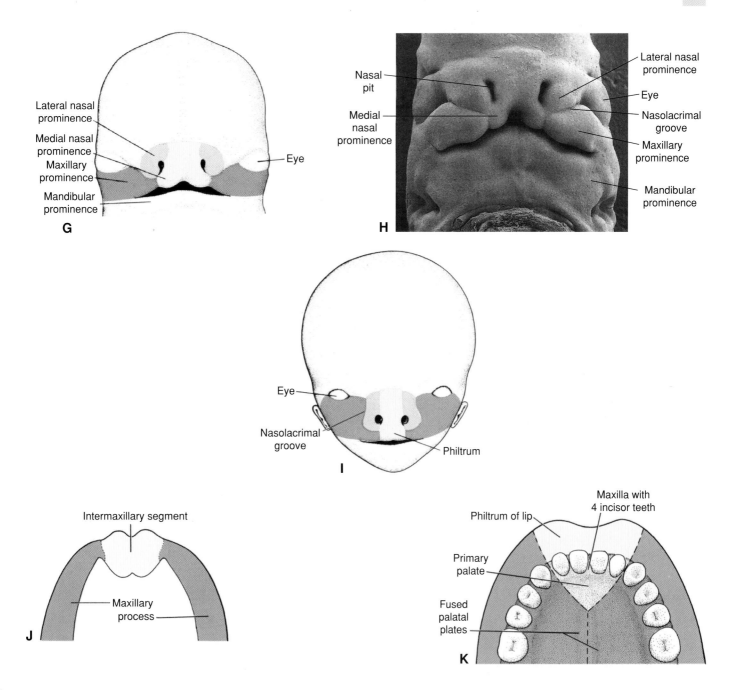

FIGURE 8.6. (*Continued*) By 7 weeks, these maxillary prominences fuse with the medial nasal prominences, which, in turn, merge in the midline (**G** and **H**). At 10 weeks, this merger is complete, such that the medial nasal prominences form the **philtrum** and the maxillary prominences form the remainder of the **upper lip** (**I**). The entire **lower lip** and **jaw** are formed by merger of the mandibular prominences across the midline (**C, F,** and **H**). Meanwhile, the **nose** is formed from five prominences: the frontonasal prominence provides the **bridge**; the medial nasal prominences give rise to the **crest** and **tip**; and the lateral nasal prominences form the **sides** (**alae**; **G–I**). The **nasal septum** is formed by proliferation of mesoderm from the frontonasal and medial nasal prominences. The **nasolacrimal duct** also forms at this time as a proliferation of ectoderm in the **nasolacrimal groove**. This groove lies between the maxillary and lateral nasal prominences and extends to the corner of the eye (**H**). In addition to forming the upper lip, the medial nasal prominences and maxillary prominences form the **upper jaw**. The medial nasal prominences contribute the **intermaxillary segment** that includes the **philtrum**; the upper jaw component containing the **4 incisor teeth**; and the **primary palate** (**J**). Maxillary prominences form the remainder of the upper jaw and the **secondary palate** (**K**).

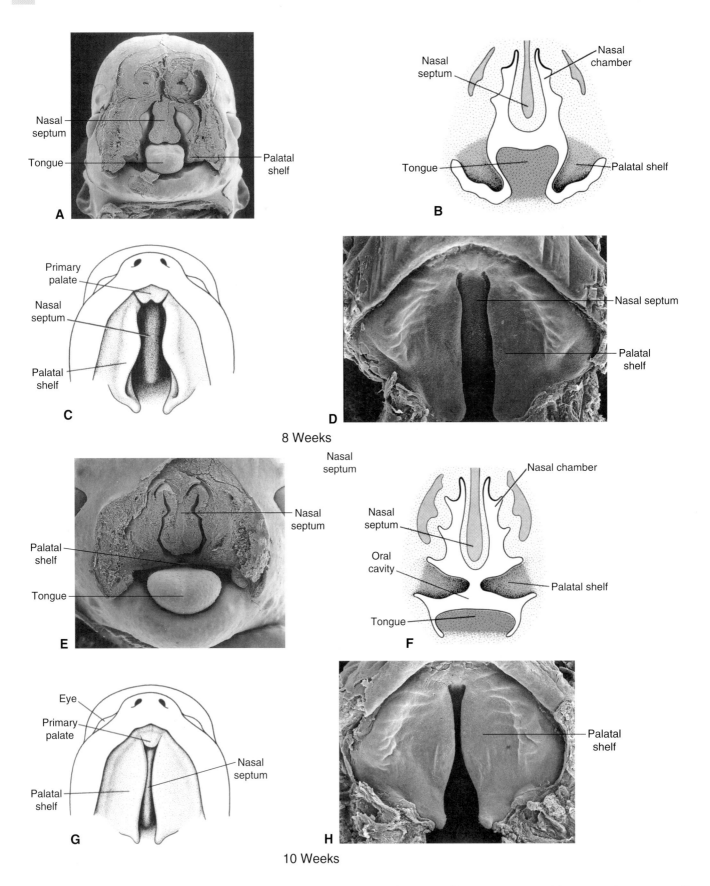

FIGURE 8.7.   The **secondary palate** develops from two extensions of the maxillary prominences that grow down vertically into the oral cavity on both sides of the developing tongue to form the **palatal shelves** in the 7th week (**A–D**). During the 8th week, the mandible grows sufficiently that the tongue "drops" and the palatal shelves "flip up" into a horizontal position above the tongue (**E–H**).   (continued)

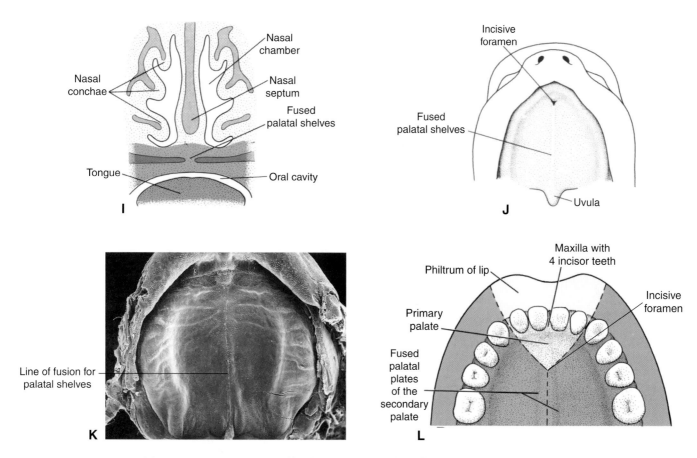

Table 8.3. **Structures Contributing to Formation of the Face and Palate**

Prominence*	Derivatives
Frontonasal	Forehead, bridge of nose, medial and lateral nasal prominences
Maxillary	Cheeks, lateral portion of the upper lip, secondary palate (palatal shelves), lateral portion of the upper jaw
Medial nasal	Philtrum of the upper lip, primary palate, upper jaw containing four incisor teeth (intermaxillary segment)
Lateral nasal	Alae (sides) of the nose
Mandibular	Lower lip and jaw

*The frontonasal prominence is a single unpaired structure; the other prominences are paired.

FIGURE 8.7. (*Continued*) In the 10th week, the palatal shelves grow together and fuse in the midline to form the **secondary palate (I–K)**. They also merge with the **primary palate**, leaving the **incisive foramen** in the midline (**J** and **L**). Table 8.3 summarizes the facial prominences and their derivatives.

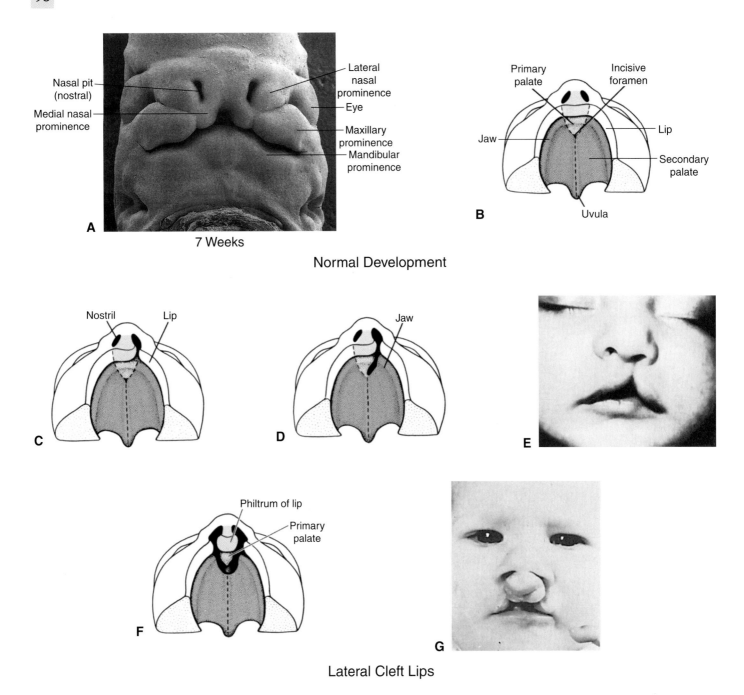

Normal Development

Lateral Cleft Lips

FIGURE 8.8. An examination of the lines of fusion and merging among the facial prominences reveals the position of facial clefts that can occur (**A** and **B**). For example, a lack of fusion between the maxillary prominence and medial nasal prominence on one side results in a **lateral cleft lip** that may or may not extend into the upper jaw and primary palate (**C–E**). If fusion fails on both sides, then **bilateral clefts** form (**F** and **G**).   (continued)

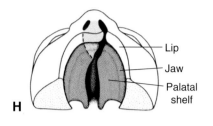

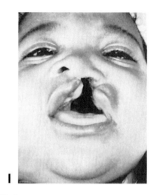

Cleft Lip with Cleft Palate

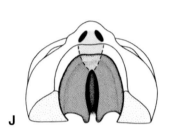

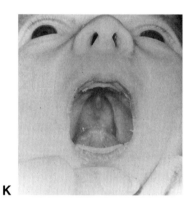

Isolated Cleft Palate

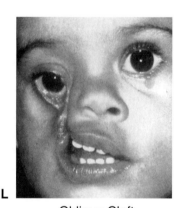

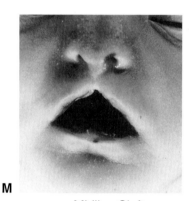

Oblique Cleft   Midline Cleft

FIGURE 8.8. (*Continued*) **Lateral clefts of the lip** (with or without cleft palate) result from failure of fusion between maxillary prominences and medial nasal prominences, are relatively common (1 per 1,000 births) and are more likely to occur (80%) in males. Isolated **cleft palate**, resulting from failure of the palatal shelves of the maxillary prominences to meet in the midline, occurs less frequently than cleft lip (1 per 2,500 births) and is more common in females (67%). The two defects often occur together. Each may be caused by teratogens, such as retinoids (e.g., Accutane), antiseizure medications (e.g., diphenylhydantoin), and corticosteroids. Others may be due to genetic abnormalities or gene–teratogen interactions (multifactorial causes; **H–K**). Failure of the nasolacrimal duct to close results in an **oblique facial cleft** (**L**), whereas failure of the medial nasal prominences to merge creates a **midline cleft** (**M**). Midline clefts often are associated with mental retardation because of the concurrent loss of midline tissue in the brain, a condition called holoprosencephaly (see Fig. 9.11C). All of these clefting defects also may arise in conjunction with other birth defects, especially cardiac abnormalities, because neural crest cells play a prominent role in morphogenesis of all of these structures.

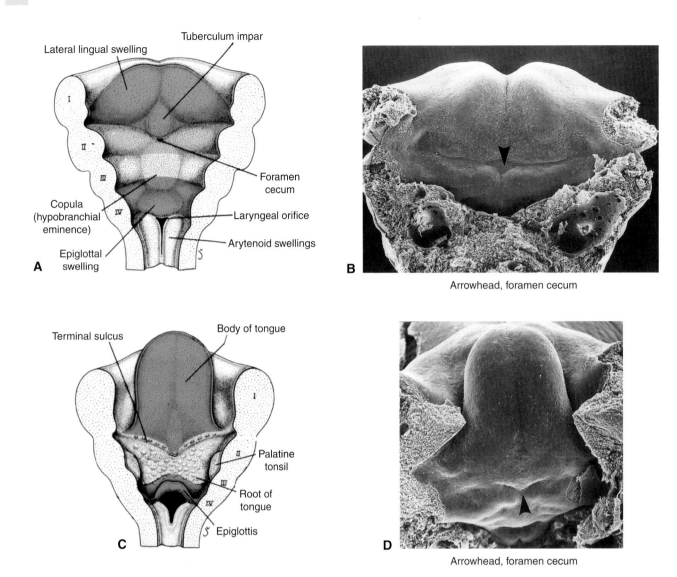

Arrowhead, foramen cecum

Arrowhead, foramen cecum

FIGURE 8.9. Like many other structures, the **tongue** begins its development at the end of the 4th week. Growth of the arches in the floor of the pharynx creates a series of swellings: the 1st arch contributes the **lateral lingual swellings** and the **tuberculum impar**; the 2nd, 3rd, and part of the 4th arch form the **copula** or **hypobranchial eminence**; and the remainder of the 4th arch gives rise to the **epiglottal swelling**, which is just cranial to the laryngeal orifice (**A** and **B**). During the next several weeks, the lateral lingual swellings grow over the tuberculum impar and form the **anterior two thirds** of the tongue, the area called the **body** of the tongue. Meanwhile, the 3rd arch overgrows the contributions of the 2nd and 4th arches, such that it forms the **posterior one third** of the tongue, called the **root**, which is delineated from the body by the **terminal sulcus** (**C** and **D**). Sensory innervation to the anterior two thirds of the tongue is via the **mandibular branch of the trigeminal nerve (the nerve of the 1st arch)**, while that to the posterior one third is by the **glossopharyngeal nerve (the nerve of the 3rd arch)**, reflecting the arches of origin for the tongue (see Table 8.1). Tongue musculature is derived from occipital somites and so is innervated by the **hypoglossal nerve**.

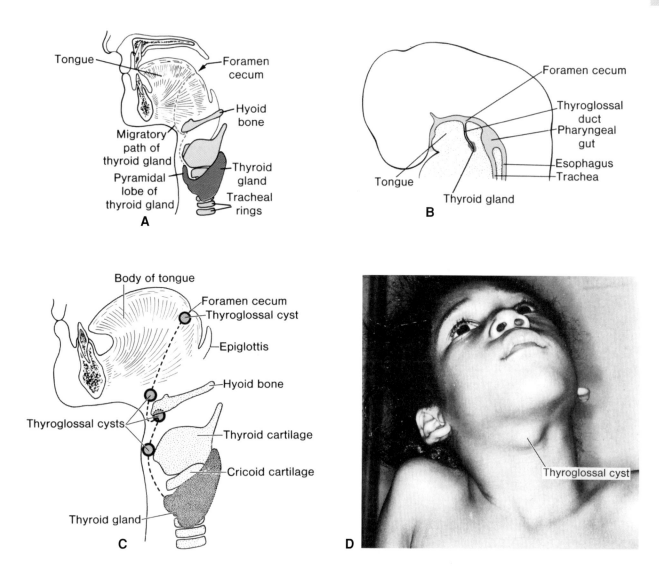

FIGURE 8.10. As the two parts of the tongue are developing and before they merge, the **thyroid gland** appears as a proliferation of **endoderm** in the midline between the tuberculum impar and copula at the site of the foramen cecum (**A**; see Fig. 8.9C). Subsequently, this endodermal bud (similar to organs forming from buds off the foregut; see Fig. 6.1) grows ventrally to form the **thyroglossal duct**, which later degenerates (**B**). Thyroid tissue at the end of the bud proliferates and continues to migrate ventrally in the midline, anterior to the hyoid bone and thyroid cartilage, to its final position in the neck (**A**). This manner of development explains why **aberrant thyroid tissue** may be found anywhere along the path of the gland's migration (**A** and **C**). Also, if the thyroglossal duct fails to pinch off and degenerate, **thyroglossal cysts** may form from its remnants (**C** and **D**).

CHAPTER 9
Central Nervous System

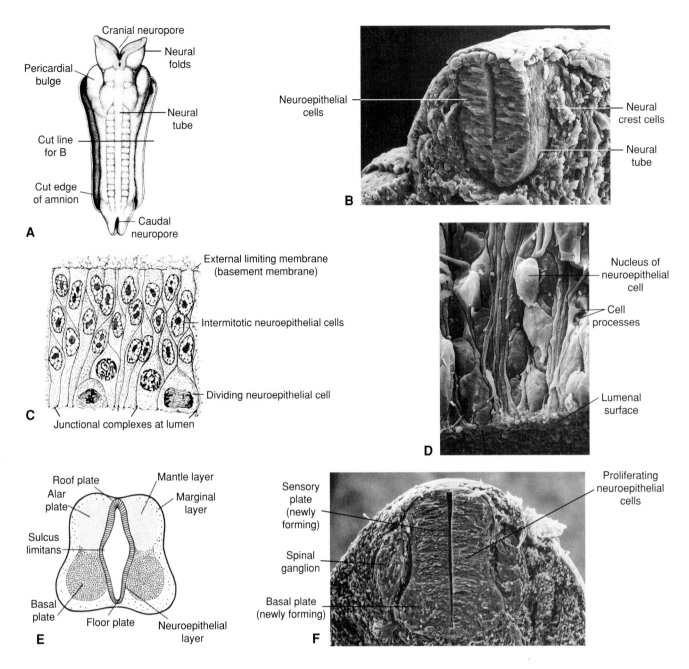

FIGURE 9.1. The **neural tube** forms the **brain** and **spinal cord**, with differentiation of the components of these two structures beginning prior to closure of the neural tube at the end of the 4th week (**A**). Initially, the wall of the **neural folds** consists of a pseudostratified layer of **neuroepithelial cells** called the **ventricular layer**. These cells are undifferentiated and rapidly proliferating. After neural tube closure, neuroepithelial cells line the lumen as a thick layer of pseudostratified epithelium, with each cell extending from the basal lamina at the external limiting membrane to the lumen (**A–D**). Nuclei of these cells move from the basal area to the luminal surface and back again, a process called **interkinetic nuclear migration**, as they pass through the stages of mitosis (**C and D**). Once nuclei reach the lumen, their cells lose their attachment to the basal membrane, and cell division occurs (**C**). Reattachment to the basal lamina then takes place, and the nuclear migration cycle starts again. After a specified number of divisions, some cells exit the proliferating population, remain close to the basal lamina, and differentiate into **neuroblasts**, **glioblasts** (supporting cells), and **oligodendroglia** (myelin-forming cells). Once differentiated cell types appear, they are organized into specific regions that extend throughout the brain and spinal cord. Thus, the **mantle layer** contains neuroblasts and forms outside the ventricular layer of proliferating cells, while the **marginal layer** lies at the periphery and contains nerve fibers (**E and F**). Eventually, the mantle layer forms **gray matter**, the marginal layer forms **white matter** (because of the myelin that covers the nerve fibers), and the ventricular layer differentiates into **ependymal cells** that line the cerebral ventricles and the lumen of the spinal cord. Later, as more and more neuroblasts accumulate, **dorsal** and **ventral thickenings** appear in the mantle layer. Dorsal thickenings form the **alar (sensory) plates**, and **ventral thickenings** form the **basal (motor) plates** (**E and F**). Thin **roof** and **floor plates** also form and serve as pathways for nerve fibers crossing from one side to the other (**E and F**). This pattern is established throughout the neural tube, although the forebrain may not have a floor plate and does not have well-developed basal plates (Fig. 9.3B).

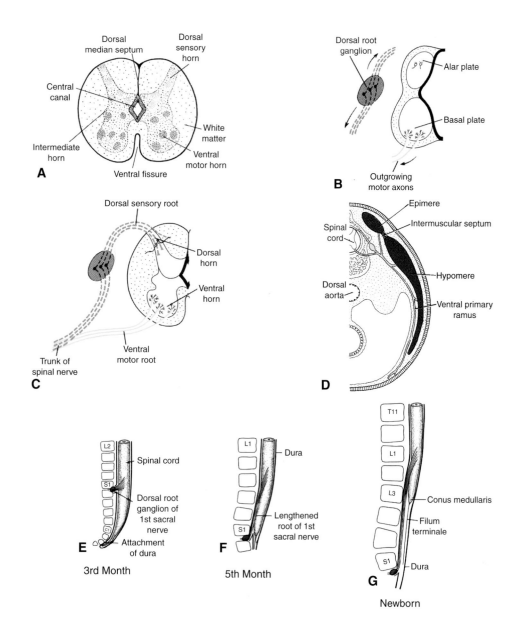

FIGURE 9.2. In the spinal cord, **alar** and **basal plates** are organized into the **dorsal (sensory)** and **ventral (motor) horns** (**A**). In addition, a **lateral (intermediate) horn** containing neurons of the **sympathetic system** (see Fig. 9.9) that develops between the dorsal and ventral horns from spinal cord segments T1 to L2 (**A**). **Spinal nerves** begin to develop in the 6th week. Fibers originating from ventral motor horn cells form **ventral (motor) roots** of the spinal nerves, while **dorsal (sensory) roots** develop from fibers of neurons whose cell bodies are located in **spinal ganglia** just lateral to the spinal cord (spinal ganglia are derived from neural crest cells; **B** and **C**). These fibers enter the cord through the dorsal (sensory) horn. Distal processes from spinal ganglia neurons join ventral roots to form spinal nerves (**C**). These nerves are very short and barely traverse the intervertebral foramina through which they pass before they divide into **dorsal** and **ventral primary rami** supplying muscles of the **epimere** and **hypomere**, respectively (**D**), as well as the skin (dermatomes) over these regions. These branches are mixed nerves, because they carry both motor and sensory fibers. At 12 weeks, each spinal nerve is aligned horizontally with the intervertebral foramina through which it exits (**E**). However, after this stage, the vertebral column grows faster than the spinal cord so that spinal nerves exit at lower and lower levels from the site of origin of their dorsal and ventral roots (**E–G**). Consequently, the dorsal and ventral roots must travel greater distances caudally to form their corresponding spinal nerve. At birth, the spinal cord of a full-term infant ends at L2-L3, whereas the dural sac and subarachnoid space extend to S2 (**G**). The pia mater, which covers the spinal cord tightly, sends an extension, the **filum terminale**, caudally from the end of the cord, the **conus medullaris**, to the coccyx (**G**). This extension marks the line of "regression" of the cord as the vertebral column grows. The many dorsal and ventral roots extending caudal to the end of the cord are called the **cauda equina (horse's tail)**. Because the cord ends at L2-3 while the subarachnoid space extends to S2, spinal taps to obtain spinal fluid for analysis can be made safely at the level of L4-5 without fear of contacting the cord. Coverings of the neural tube include the dura mater (outer layer), which arises from surrounding mesoderm, and the pia (innermost layer) and arachnoid (middle layer), which are derived from neural crest cells.

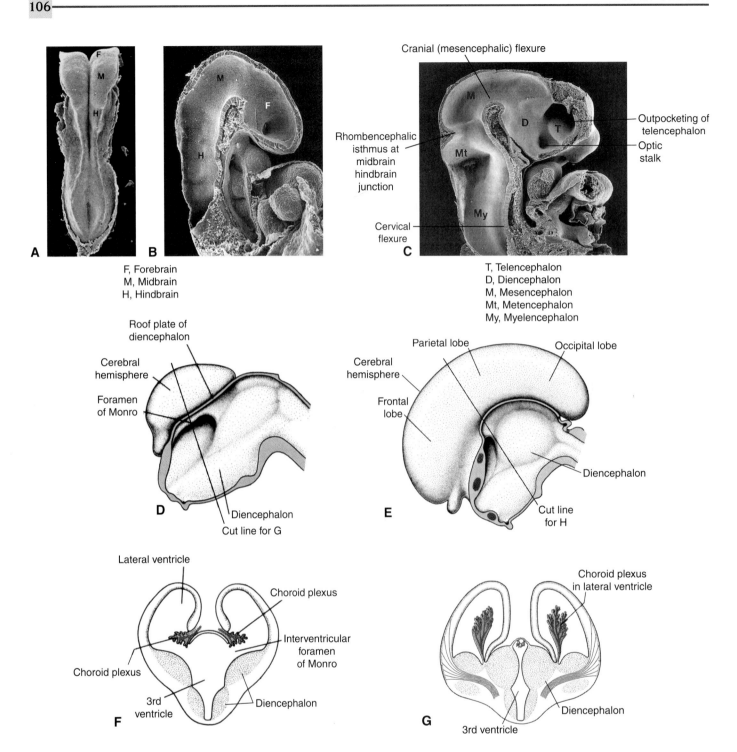

F, Forebrain
M, Midbrain
H, Hindbrain

Cranial (mesencephalic) flexure

Rhombencephalic
isthmus at
midbrain
hindbrain
junction

Outpocketing of
telencephalon

Optic
stalk

Cervical
flexure

T, Telencephalon
D, Diencephalon
M, Mesencephalon
Mt, Metencephalon
My, Myelencephalon

Roof plate of
diencephalon

Cerebral
hemisphere

Foramen
of Monro

Diencephalon

Cut line for G

Parietal lobe

Occipital lobe

Cerebral
hemisphere

Frontal
lobe

Diencephalon

Cut line
for H

Lateral ventricle

Choroid plexus

Interventricular
foramen
of Monro

Choroid plexus

3rd
ventricle

Diencephalon

Choroid plexus
in lateral ventricle

Diencephalon

3rd ventricle

FIGURE 9.3. As with the spinal cord region, differentiation of the **brain** begins prior to closure of the neural tube. Thus, during cranial neural fold formation and elevation, three primary brain regions, the **prosencephalon (forebrain), mesencephalon (midbrain),** and **rhombencephalon (hindbrain)** initiate their development (**A**). Then, once neural tube closure is completed in the 4th week, these regions form the three **primary brain vesicles** (**B**). During the 5th week, these vesicles differentiate into five parts of the brain (**C**). Thus, the prosencephalon forms the **telencephalon** and **diencephalon**; the mesencephalon does not subdivide; and the rhombencephalon forms the **metencephalon** and **myelencephalon (medulla oblongata)**. Formation of these vesicles causes the brain to lengthen and bend, creating the **cervical** and **cranial (mesencephalic) flexures** (**C**). As differentiation of these brain vesicles continues, they become organized into **alar (sensory) plates** dorsally and **basal (motor) plates** ventrally and also develop **roof** and **floor plates**. However, in the telencephalon and diencephalon, alar plates predominate and basal plates regress. The telencephalon forms the **cerebral hemispheres**, which arise as outpocketings from the prosencephalon (**C**) and expand to cover most of the other brain regions (**D** and **E**). Cavities in the hemispheres form the **lateral ventricles**, and these communicate with the cavity of the diencephalon, the **3rd ventricle**, via the **interventricular foramina of Monro** (**F** and **G**). Each hemisphere also contains a **choroid plexus**, a richly vascularized proliferation of the pia, that produces **cerebrospinal fluid** (**F** and **G**). (continued)

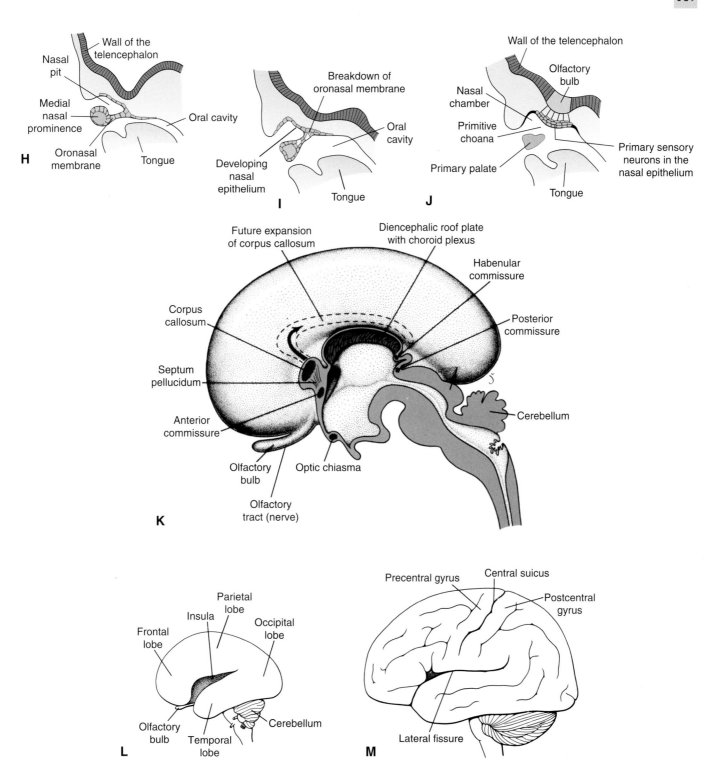

FIGURE 9.3. *(Continued)* **Olfactory bulbs** develop on the floor of the anterior portion of the cerebral hemispheres during the 6th week (**E** and **H–J**). At the same time, ectoderm cells in the **nasal placode** (see Fig. 8.6) begin to differentiate into primary sensory neurons in the nasal epithelium. By the 7th week, these neurons grow toward and contact secondary neurons in the olfactory bulbs (**J**). The bulbs and tracts of the secondary neurons lengthen to form the **olfactory nerve** (**K**). In addition, numerous cross-connecting pathways called **commissures** are established between the hemispheres (**K**), and the **optic chiasma** also forms a commissure in the diencephalon. By 7 months, the cerebral hemispheres cover most of the rest of the brain and have a smooth surface (**L**). During the last 2 months gestation, the surface of the hemispheres grows so rapidly that many **gyri** (convolutions) form, separated by **fissures** and **sulci** (**M**). The **cerebral cortex** develops in these hemispheres.

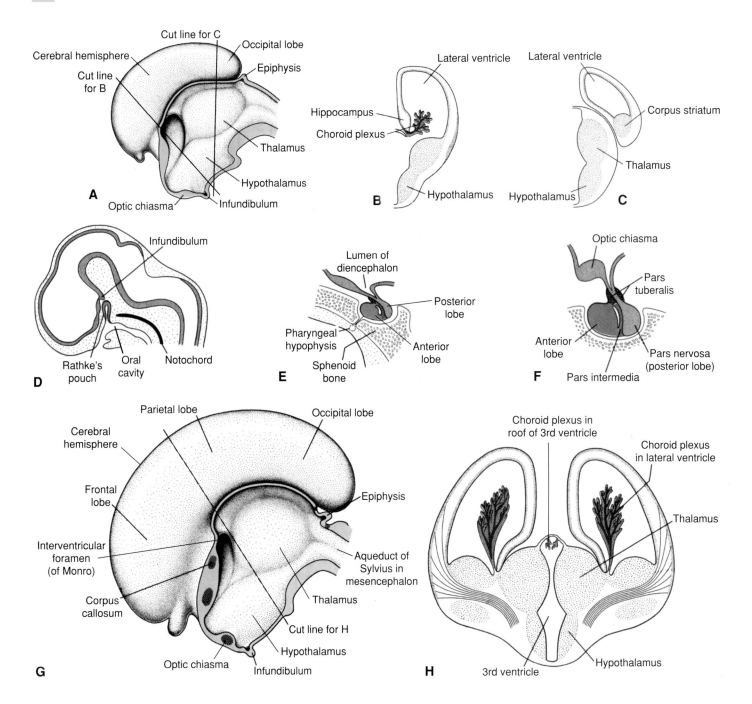

FIGURE 9.4. The **diencephalon** forms the **optic stalk** (which becomes the **optic nerve**) and **cup**, part of the **hypophysis (pituitary gland), thalamus, hypothalamus,** and **epiphysis (A–C).** The **epiphysis** forms from the roof plate as an epithelial evagination in the 7th week (**A**). Here it serves as a receptor for changes in daylight and darkness that affect endocrine and hormonal rhythms. The **posterior lobe** of the pituitary forms from a ventral extension of diencephalic ectoderm called the **infundibulum.** The infundibulum forms the **stalk** and the **pars nervosa (posterior lobe)** of the pituitary gland (**D–F**). The **anterior lobe,** or **adenohypophysis,** develops from an outpocketing of ectoderm called **Rathke's pouch** that forms in the roof of the oral cavity, in front of the **buccopharyngeal membrane (D).** This pouch grows dorsally toward the infundibulum, pinches off from the oral cavity, and assumes a position immediately anterior to the posterior lobe (**E**). In addition, a small dorsal extension of this pouch, the **pars tuberalis,** grows to surround the stalk of the pituitary, while an outpocketing from its posterior wall forms the **pars intermedia (F).** Occasionally, Rathke's pouch fails to pinch off. This failure results in pituitary tissue in the roof of the pharynx, a condition called a **pharyngeal hypophysis (E).** The lumen of the diencephalon forms the **3rd ventricle,** which also has a **choroid plexus (G and H).** This ventricle communicates with the lateral ventricles in the cerebral hemispheres through the **interventricular foramina of Monro** and with the mesencephalon via the **aqueduct of Sylvius (G).**

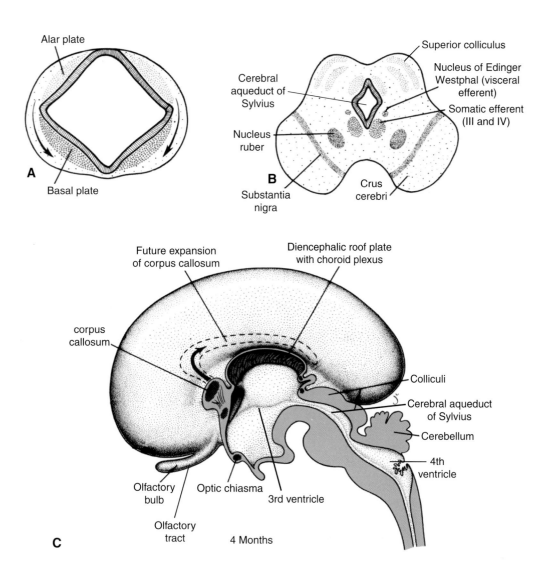

FIGURE 9.5. The **mesencephalon** has well-defined basal, alar, roof, and floor plates (**A**). The basal plates form **motor nuclei** for the **oculomotor (CN III)** and **trochlear (CN IV)** nerves and for the **sphincter pupillary muscle** (the **nucleus of Edinger Westphal**; **B**). The marginal layer in the basal plate region differentiates into the **crux cerebri**, which serve as pathways for descending fibers from the cerebral cortex (**B**). Meanwhile, the alar region forms nuclei that migrate ventrally to form the **red nucleus** and the **substantia nigra** (**A**, *arrows*, and **B**). It also forms nuclei that migrate dorsally into the roof plate to form the **anterior (superior)** and **posterior (inferior) colliculi**, which serve as synaptic relay stations for **visual** and **auditory signals**, respectively (**B** and **C**). The lumen of the mesencephalon is the **aqueduct of Sylvius** that connects the 3rd and 4th ventricles (**B** and **C**).

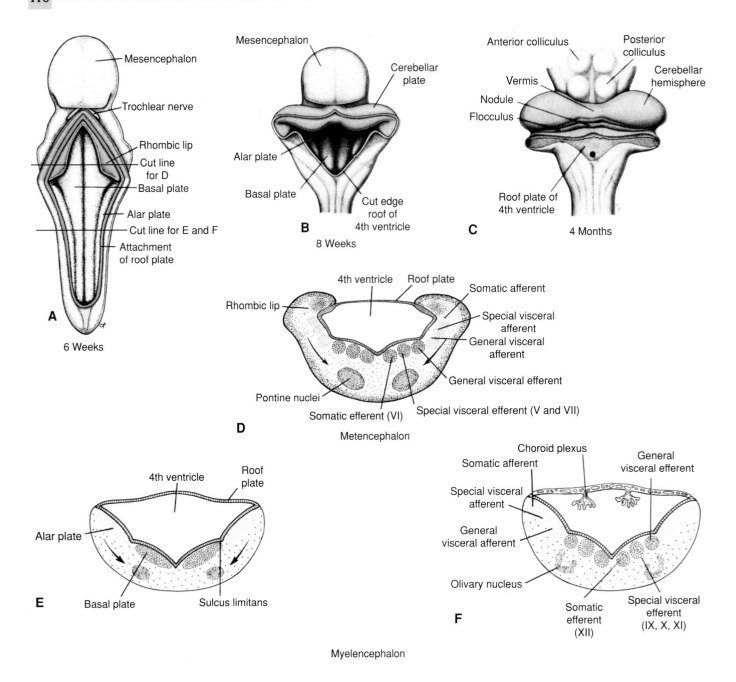

A 6 Weeks

B 8 Weeks

C 4 Months

D Metencephalon

E Myelencephalon

F

FIGURE 9.6. The **metencephalon** forms the **cerebellum**, a coordination center for posture and movement, from its alar plate region. Initially, the dorsolateral parts of these alar plates grow medially to form the rhombic lips (**A**). By 8 weeks, these lips expand to form the **cerebellar plate** (**B**), and by 12 weeks this plate gives rise to two **cerebellar hemispheres** and a **midline vermis** (**C**). Transverse fissures then appear and separate another segment with symmetrical lateral parts called **flocculi** and a central part called the **nodule** (**C**). Together these parts constitute the **flocculonodular lobe**. The alar plate also forms nuclei for sensory nerves as well as the **pontine nuclei** that migrate ventrally into the basal plates (**D**, *arrows*). The basal plate of the metencephalon forms the **pons (bridge)**, which carries nerve fibers connecting the cerebral cortex and cerebellum with the spinal cord. It also forms motor nuclei for the **abducens (CN VI)** nerve and for the special visceral efferent components (supplying muscles derived from pharyngeal arches; Table 9.1) of the **mandibular (CN V)** and **facial (CN VII) nerves** (**D**). The lumen of the metencephalon is part of the fourth ventricle, which communicates with the cerebral aqueduct of Sylvius (**D**). The **myelencephalon** has everted walls and a thin roof plate covering the **fourth ventricle** (**A, E,** and **F**). This roof plate consists of a single layer of ependymal cells covered by vascular mesenchyme of the pia mater (**F**). Together these layers form the **tela choroidea**. Later, the vascular mesenchyme proliferates to form the **choroid plexus** covering the fourth ventricle. The alar plates form sensory nuclei, some of which migrate ventrally to form the **olivary nucleus** (**E,** *arrows*, and **F**). Motor nuclei in the basal plates include those for the **glossopharyngeal (CN IX), vagus (CN X), spinal accessory (CN XI),** and **hypoglossal (CN XII)** nerves (**F**).

Table 9.1. Origins of Cranial Nerves and Their Composition

Cranial Nerve	Brain Region	Type	Innervation
Olfactory (I)	Telencephalon	SVA	Nasal epithelium (smell)
Optic (II)	Diencephalon	SSA	Retina (vision)
Oculomotor (III)	Mesencephalon	GSE	Sup., inf., med. rectus, inf. oblique, levator palpebrae sup. m.
		GVE (ciliary ganglion)	Sphincter pupillae, ciliary m.
Trochlear (IV)	Metencephalon (exits mesencephalon)	GSE	Sup. oblique m.
Trigeminal (V)	Metencephalon	GSA (trigeminal ganglion)	Skin, mouth, facial m., teeth, ant. two thirds of tongue
		GVA (trigeminal ganglion)	Proprioception: skin, muscles, joints
		SVE (branchiomotor)	M. of mastication, mylohyoid, ant. belly of digastric, tensor veli palati, post. belly of digastric m.
Abducens (VI)	Metencephalon	GSE	Lateral rectus m.
Facial (VII)	Metencephalon	SVA (geniculate ganglion)	Taste ant. two thirds of tongue
		GSA (geniculate ganglion)	Skin ext. auditory meatus
		GVA (geniculate ganglion)	Ant. two thirds of tongue
		SVE (branchiomotor)	M. of facial expression, stapedius, stylohyoid, post. belly of digastric
		GVE (pterygopalatine and submandibular ganglia)	Submandibular, sublingual, and lacrimal glands
Vestibulocochlear (VIII)	Metencephalon	SSA (vestibular and spiral ganglia)	Semicircular canals, utricle, saccule (balance)
			Spiral organ of Corti (hearing)
Glossopharyngeal (IX)	Myelencephalon	SVA (inferior ganglion)	Post. one third of tongue (taste)
		GVA (superior ganglion)	Parotid gland, carotid body and sinus, middle ear
		GSA (inferior ganglion)	External ear
		SVE (branchiomotor)	Stylopharyngeus
		GVE (otic ganglion)	Parotid gland
Vagus (X)	Myelencephalon	SVA (inferior ganglion)	Palate and epiglottis (taste)
		GVA (superior ganglion)	Base of tongue, pharynx, larynx, trachea, heart, esophagus, stomach, intestines
		GSA (superior ganglion)	External auditory meatus
		SVE (branchiomotor)	Constrictor m. pharynx, intrinsic m. larynx, sup. two thirds esophagus
		GVE (ganglia at or near viscera)	Trachea, bronchi, digestive tract, heart
Spinal accessory (XI)	Myelencephalon	SVE (branchiomotor)	Strenocleidomastoid, trapezius m.
		GSE	Soft palate, pharynx (with X)
Hypoglossal (XII)	Myelencephalon	GSE	M. of tongue (except palatoglossus)

GSA, general somatic afferent (parasympathetics); GSE, general somatic efferent; GVA, general visceral afferent; GVE, general visceral efferent; SSA, special somatic afferent; SVA, special visceral afferent; SVE, special visceral efferent.

ant., anterior; inf., inferior; m., muscle; med., medial; post., posterior; sup., superior.

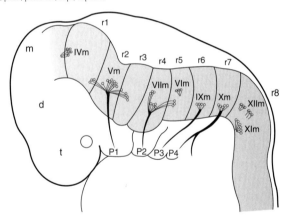

FIGURE 9.7. By the 5th week, the brain can be divided into the **brainstem**, which includes the mesencephalon, metencephalon, and myelencephalon, and the **higher centers**, including the cerebellum (derived from the metencephalon) and derivatives of the forebrain (e.g., cerebral hemispheres, thalamus, hypothalamus). At this time, nuclei for all of the **cranial nerves** (**CN**; see Table 9.1) are present, and all but two (the olfactory and optic) are located in the brainstem. Here their alar and basal nuclei are organized into seven **columns**, described individually in this paragraph, that serve motor and sensory functions (see Figs. 9.5B and 9.6D and F). (1) The **somatic efferent column** supplies extrinsic eye muscles (CN III, IV, and VI) and muscles of the tongue (CN XII). (2) The **special visceral efferent column** supplies muscles derived from the pharyngeal arches (CN V, VII, IX, X, and XI). Because it serves muscles of the pharyngeal arches, which in the past were called branchial (gill) arches, this column sometimes is called the **branchiomotor column**. The **spinal accessory nerve** (CN XI) is included in this group because its nucleus is located in this column, not because the muscles it innervates—the sternocleidomastoid and trapezius—are derived from pharyngeal arches. (3) The **visceral efferent column** supplies the sphincter pupillary and ciliary muscles (CN III), the submandibular and lacrimal glands (CN VII), the parotid gland (CN IX), and the viscera (CN X). (4) The **visceral afferent column** receives input from the parotid gland, carotid body, and middle ear (CN IX) and the viscera (CN X). (5) The **special visceral afferent** column receives taste impulses via CN VII (the anterior two thirds of the tongue), CN IX (the posterior third of the tongue), and CN X (the palate and epiglottis). (6) The **general afferent column** receives general sensation impulses from the face (CN V and VII) and from the nasal, oral, pharyngeal, and laryngeal regions (CN V, IX, and X). (7) The **special somatic afferent** column is associated with hearing and balance (CN VIII).

Table 9.2. **Contributions of Neural Crest Cells and Placodes to Ganglia of the Cranial Nerves**

Nerve	Ganglion	Origin
Oculomotor (III)	Ciliary (visceral efferent)	Neural crest at forebrain–midbrain junction
Trigeminal (V)	Trigeminal (general afferent)	Neural crest at forebrain–midbrain junction, trigeminal placode
Facial (VII)	Superior (general and special afferent)	Hindbrain neural crest, first epibranchial placode
	Inferior (geniculate; general and special afferent)	First epibranchial placode
		Hindbrain neural crest
	Sphenopalatine (visceral efferent)	Hindbrain neural crest
	Submandibular (visceral efferent)	
Vestibulocochlear (VIII)	Acoustic (cochlear; special afferent)	Otic placode
	Vestibular (special afferent)	Otic placode, hindbrain neural crest
Glossopharyngeal (IX)	Superior (general and special afferent)	Hindbrain neural crest
	Inferior (petrosal; general and special afferent)	Second epibranchial placode
	Otic (visceral efferent)	Hindbrain neural crest
Vagus (X)	Superior (general afferent)	Hindbrain neural crest
	Inferior (nodose; general and special afferent)	Hindbrain neural crest; third, fourth epibranchial placodes
	Vagal parasympathetic (visceral efferent)	Hindbrain neural crest

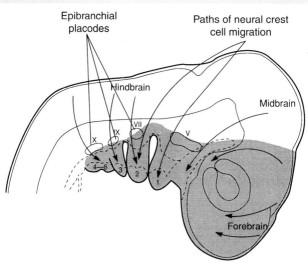

FIGURE 9.8. **Sensory ganglia** for cranial nerves form outside of the brain (a situation analogous to spinal ganglia outside the spinal cord). These are derived from **ectodermal placodes** and **neural crest cells** (Table 9.2). Placodes include the **nasal, otic**, and **four epibranchial placodes** that lie dorsal to the pharyngeal arches. Epibranchial placodes contribute to ganglia for nerves of the pharyngeal arches (cranial nerves V, VII, IX and X).

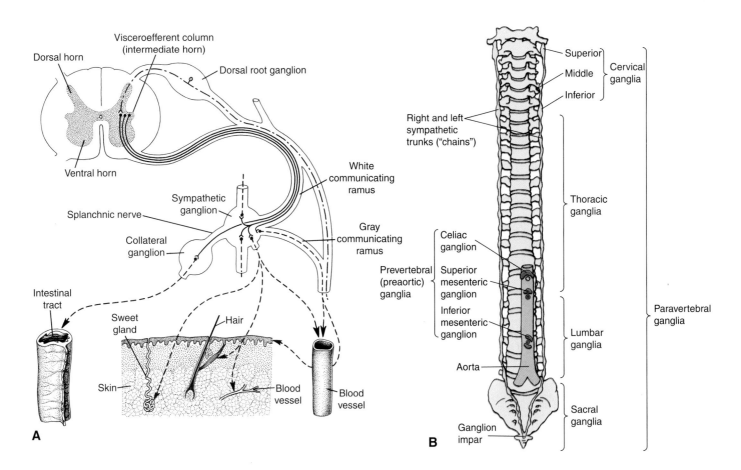

FIGURE 9.9. The **autonomic nervous system** is divided into two parts: the **sympathetic** and **parasympathetic systems**. The sympathetic system originates in the **viscereofferent column (intermediate horn)** of the spinal cord from thoracic (T1) to lumbar (L2) segments (**A**). Neurons in this column send **preganglionic sympathetic fibers** with spinal nerves from T1-L2 to the **sympathetic trunk** via **white rami communicantes** (**A**). The sympathetic trunks consist of a chain of ganglia that are formed from neural crest cells in the 5th week and are interconnected by longitudinal fibers. The chain is located lateral to the vertebral bodies along the posterior body wall and extends from sacral to cervical regions (**B**). Preganglionic fibers, arriving in the chain, may synapse with ganglia at their level of entry; or they may turn to synapse on ganglia cranial or caudal to their level of entry; or they may pass directly through the trunks to synapse in additional sympathetic ganglia around the aorta (**A** and **B**). These ganglia are called **collateral** or **preaortic ganglia** and form **plexuses** around the major aortic vessels, i.e. the **celiac** and **mesenteric plexuses** (**B**). Preganglionic fibers that pass directly through the trunks form the **splanchnic nerves—greater (T5-T9), lesser (T10-T11), least (T12),** and **lumbar (L1-L2)**—serving the gut (**A**). **Postganglionic fibers** leaving the sympathetic trunks form **gray rami communicantes** as they rejoin each spinal nerve (**A**). Postganglionic fibers from collateral ganglia pass directly to the organs they serve. Note that white rami communicantes are present only at levels T1 to L2, reflecting the site of origin of their nerve cell bodies, whereas gray rami exist at all spinal cord levels. White rami have a myelin covering that gives them their white appearance, but gray rami are unmyelinated. The **parasympathetic system** originates in the **brainstem** (associated with CN III, VII, IX, and X; see Table 9.1) and **sacral segments** (S2-S4, pelvic splanchnic nerves) of the spinal cord. Preganglionic fibers synapse in ganglia located close to the organs they supply such that postganglionic parasympathetic fibers tend to be much shorter than postganglionic sympathetic fibers. Ganglia of the parasympathetic system are derived from neural crest cells. In some cases, neural crest cells fail to migrate, leaving part or all of the colon and or rectum without parasympathetic ganglia, a condition called **Hirschsprung's disease (congenital megacolon)**.

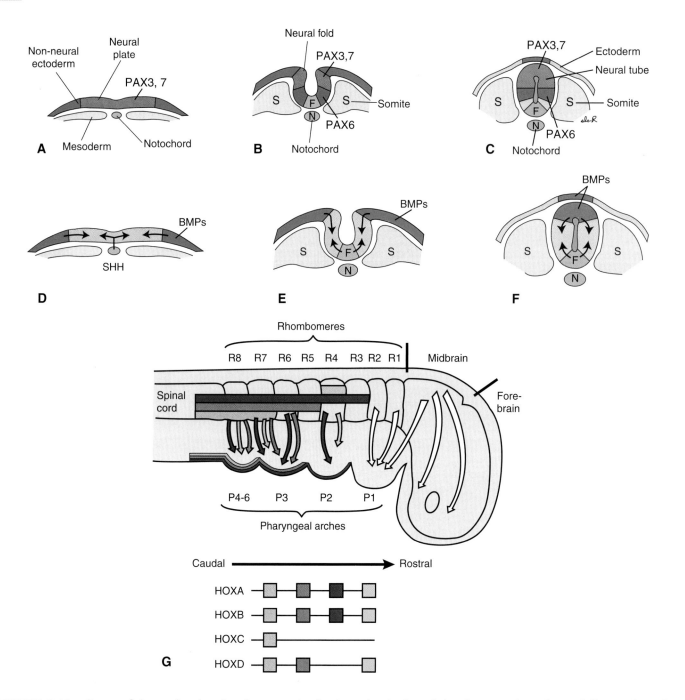

FIGURE 9.10. Some of the molecular signals patterning brain and spinal cord development have been delineated. At the neural plate stage in the 3rd week of development, the entire plate expresses the homeobox-containing genes *PAX3* and *PAX7* (**A**). As the neural folds begin to form, sonic hedgehog (SHH), secreted by the notochord (and later by the floor plate), downregulates expression of *PAX3* and *PAX7* in the midline and ventral half of the neural tube (**B–F**). This inhibition, together with a high SHH concentration, "ventralizes" the neural tube, such that this ventral region forms a floor plate and a basal plate containing motor neurons. Meanwhile, bone morphogenetic proteins (BMP4 and 7), secreted by adjacent non-neural ectoderm, maintain and upregulate *PAX3* and *PAX7* expression in the dorsal half of the neural tube, thereby stimulating formation of the alar and roof plates (**A–F**). *PAX6* also is upregulated when the neural folds form, but its role has not been determined. The **hindbrain (rhombencephalon)** is segmented into eight segments called **rhombomeres**, the identity and derivatives of which are regulated by an overlapping *HOX* code (**G**) analogous to that specifying the body axis (see Fig. 3.9B) and pharyngeal arches (see Fig. 8.3). In fact, the code for the pharyngeal arches is specified by neural crest cells that migrate to the arches from the rhombomeres, carrying the rhombomeric code with them (**G**, *arrows*). (continued)

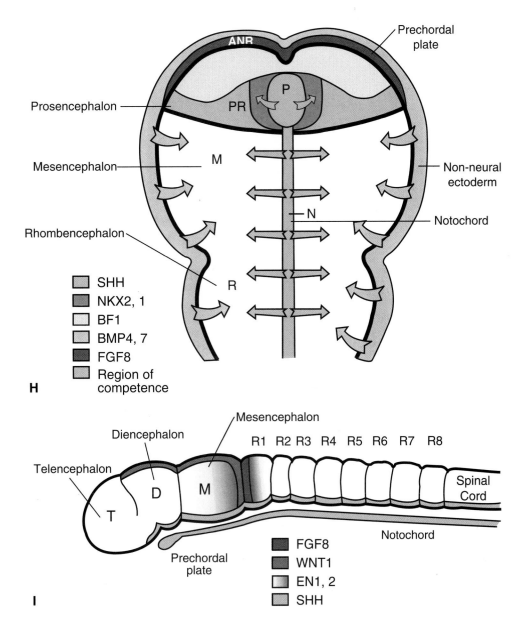

FIGURE 9.10. (*Continued*) Establishment of the fore- and midbrain boundaries depends on a different set of homeobox genes that are not of the *Antenepedia (HOX)* class. Thus, at the neural plate stage, even before neural folds form, *LIM1*, expressed in the prechordal plate, and *OTX2*, expressed in the neural plate, designate the fore- and midbrain regions. Later, once neural folds and pharyngeal arches appear, additional homeobox genes, including *OTX1*, *EMX1*, and *EMX2* are expressed in overlapping patterns to further specify the identities of these brain regions. Once the primary brain regions have been delineated at the neural plate stage, two new organizing centers appear: the anterior neural ridge (ANR), at the junction of the neural plate and non-neural ectoderm (**H**); and the isthmus, at the midbrain–hindbrain junction (**I**). At the four-somite stage, the ANR secretes fibroblast growth factor 8 (FGF8), which, in turn, induces expression of *brain factor 1 (BF1)*. *BF1* regulates development of the telencephalon. Ventral midline patterning of all the brain regions (and the spinal cord; **B**) is regulated by SHH. SHH patterns a number of structures, including the hypothalamus, the differentiation of which is regulated by *NKX2.1* expression. Dorsal and lateral patterning is signaled by bone morphogenetic proteins 4 and 7 (BMP4 and 7) secreted by non-neural ectoderm (**H**). (The same signal occurs in the spinal cord [**B**].) These proteins initiate other genetic cascades that regulate differentiation in these regions, while they repress *BF1* expression. The other regulating center, the isthmus, at the midbrain–hindbrain junction (**I**), also secretes FGF8, which induces expression of two additional homeobox genes, *EN1* and *EN2*. *EN1* regulates dorsal midbrain and anterior hindbrain (cerebellum) development; *EN2* also participates in cerebellar development. These genes are assisted in their signaling roles by the growth factor WNT1, which is also induced in this region by FGF8. R1–R8, rhombomeres.

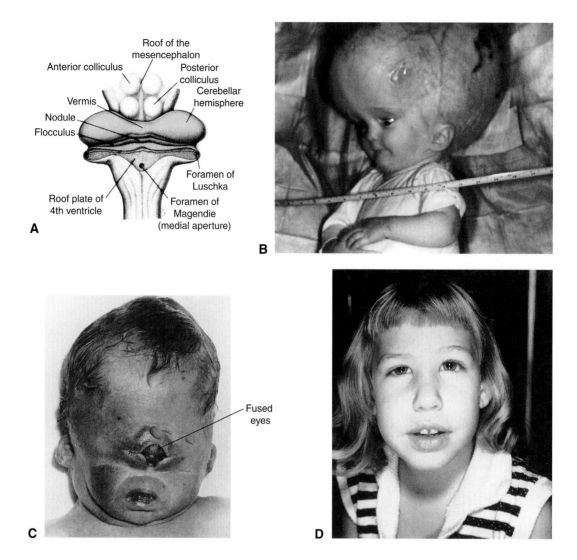

FIGURE 9.11. Birth defects involving the brain and spinal cord are common and include the neural tube defects **spina bifida** and **anencephaly**, and other related abnormalities (see Fig. 3.10). **Hydrocephaly** results when there is a blockage in the flow of **cerebrospinal fluid**. Normally, this fluid is made by the **choroid plexuses** in the **brain ventricles**, and it circulates in the lumens of the ventricles and spinal cord. Ultimately, it flows out the roof of the 4th ventricle through two lateral and one central openings called the **foramina of Luschka** and **Magendie**, respectively (**A**). From here it flows into the subarachnoid space, where it is resorbed by **arachnoid granulations** in the dural sinuses around the brain. When this circulatory pathway is impeded, fluid accumulates in the ventricles and, if the cranial sutures have not fused and if the pressure is not relieved, the head may swell considerably (**B**). The pressure can be relieved by placing a shunt to drain the fluid from a lateral ventricle to the abdomen. The site where blockage most commonly occurs is in the **cerebral aqueduct of Sylvius** in the **mesencephalon**. **Holoprosencephaly** is another brain defect that arises when there is a deficiency of midline tissue for brain and facial development. The severity of the abnormality varies, but in its worst form, there is such a loss of midline structures that there is a single cerebral hemisphere with a common ventricle, and the eyes are fused, a condition called **synophthalmia** (**C**). Holoprosencephaly also often is accompanied by **midline facial defects**, such as a **median cleft lip** or abnormalities of the nose. The severity of these defects usually can predict the severity of defects in the brain. **Mutations in SHH**, the gene that regulates midline development of the brain and spinal cord (see Fig. 9.10), are responsible for some cases, but the defect also can be produced by maternal alcohol abuse and maternal diabetes. The midline forms during the 3rd and 4th weeks of development, and this time—a time when many women do not even realize the are pregnant—is the most vulnerable period for this defect to occur. In some cases, the brain fails to grow sufficiently, resulting in a smaller than normal brain (**microcephaly**; **D**). In most cases, affected children are mentally retarded. Many other causes of mental retardation and learning disabilities exist. These conditions are often present as part of a syndrome or from exposure to a teratogen, such as alcohol (see Table 11.4). In fact, prenatal exposure to alcohol is a leading cause of mental retardation.

CHAPTER 10

Eye and Ear

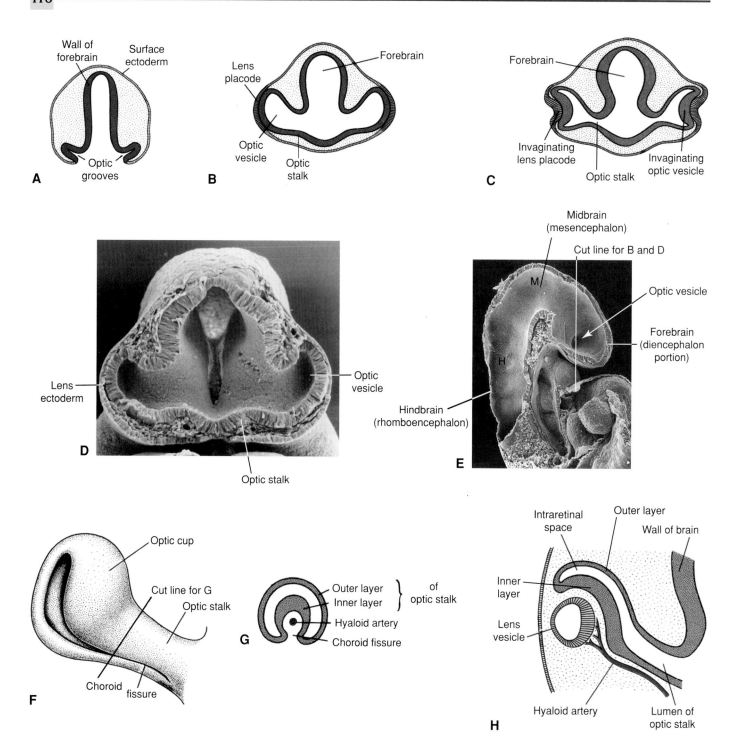

FIGURE 10.1. **Eye** development is initiated at the beginning of the 4th week when outpocketings of the **diencephalon** form (**A–E**). Eventually, these outpocketings form the **optic stalks** and **optic vesicles** (**B–E**). The vesicles grow out to contact overlying ectoderm and induce it to form the **lens** (**B–D**). Meanwhile, the outer surface of the optic vesicle and part of the stalk invaginate, and this movement creates the **optic cup** and **choroid fissure**, respectively (**C–F**). The cup itself then has inner and outer layers (**G** and **H**). The choroid fissure houses the hyaloid artery to the lens (**G** and **H**). Later, the edges of the fissure and cup fuse to form a round opening called the pupil.   (continued)

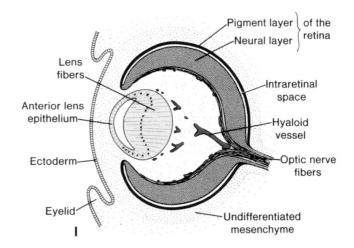

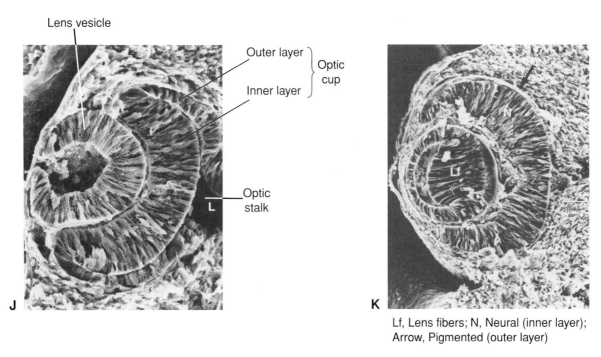

Lf, Lens fibers; N, Neural (inner layer);
Arrow, Pigmented (outer layer)

FIGURE 10.1.   (*Continued*) The outer layer of the optic cup then forms the **pigmented layer of the retina**, while the inner layer differentiates into the **neural layer** with its **rods** and **cones** (I). The lens itself forms from surface ectoderm overlying the optic cup (**B** and **D**). Once induced by the underlying cup, this ectoderm thickens to form a **placode** and then invaginates and pinches off in the 5th week to form the **lens vesicle** (**H** and **J**). During the next 2 weeks, posterior cells in the lens vesicle elongate to form **lens fibers** that eventually contact the anterior epithelial cells, thereby obliterating the lumen of the lens vesicle (**I** and **K**).

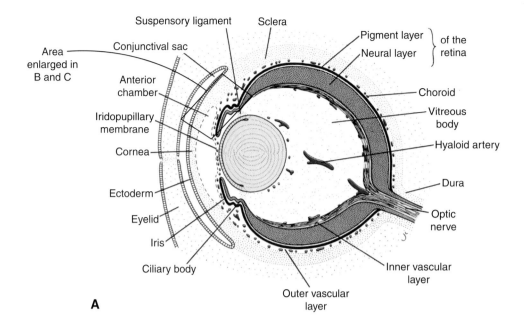

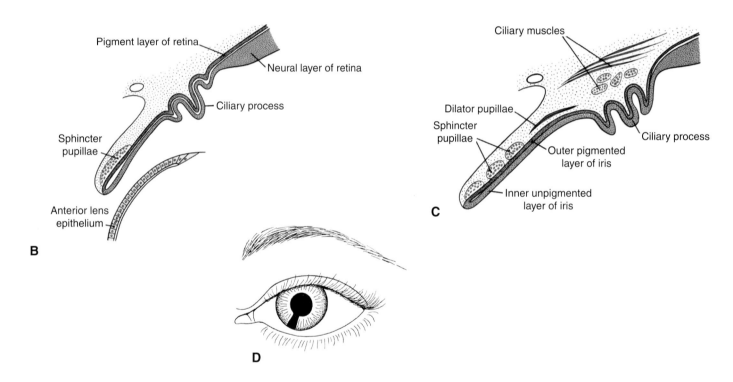

FIGURE 10.2. Mesenchyme surrounding the optic cup differentiates into the **sclera** and an outer vascular layer called the **choroid** next to the cup (**A**). Mesenchyme in front of the lens forms a cavity called the **anterior chamber**. Mesenchyme in the posterior wall of this chamber forms the **iridopupillary membrane**, which later breaks down; mesenchyme in the anterior wall forms the **cornea**, which also has an outer layer derived from ectoderm (**A**). **Eyelids** and the **conjunctival sac** form anterior to the cornea (**A**). The **vitreous chamber** forms behind the lens and fills with a gelatinous material called the **vitreous body**. The hyaloid artery within the posterior chamber degenerates and leaves the **hyaloid canal**. Meanwhile, in the 7th week, the choroid fissure closes and nerve fibers begin to fill the optic stalk as it is transformed into the **optic nerve** (**A**). In the center of the nerve fiber, the hyaloid artery becomes the **central artery to the retina**. The anterior portion of the cup forms the **iris** (including the **pupillary sphincter** and **dilator muscles**) as well as the **ciliary body** containing the **ciliary muscles** (**B** and **C**). **Suspensory ligaments** connect the ciliary body to the **lens** (**A**), such that contraction of the ciliary muscle changes tension in the ligament and controls the shape of the lens. Sometimes the choroid fissure fails to close, resulting in a **coloboma**. These defects usually involve only the iris, but may extend all the way into the optic stalk (**D**).

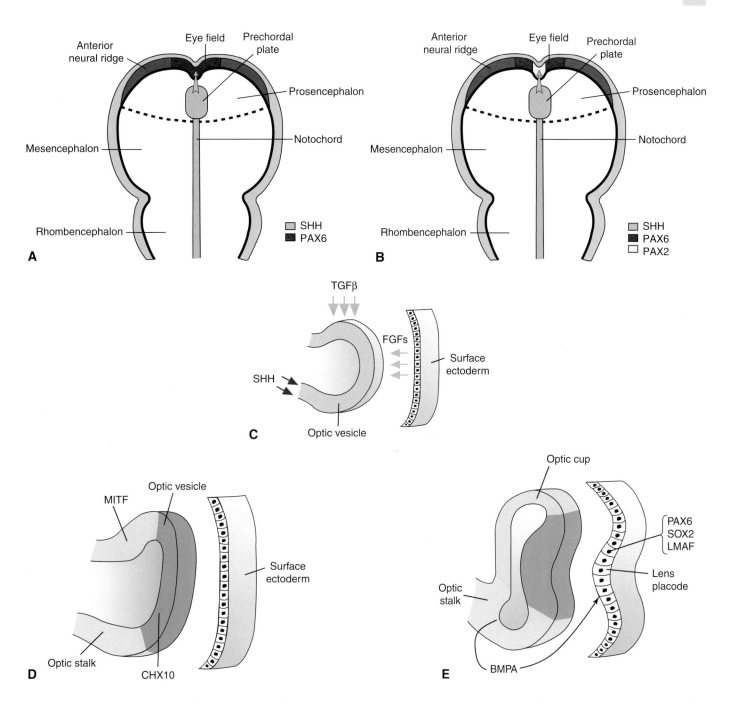

FIGURE 10.3. The transcription factor *PAX6* is the master gene for eye development. Initially, it is expressed in a band in the anterior neural ridge (**A**; ANR; see Fig. 9.10), and it defines a large, single eye field across the midline. This field is divided into two fields by expression of *sonic hedgehog (SHH)* in the midline (**A**). *SHH* expression downregulates *PAX6* expression in the midline and upregulates expression of *PAX2* (**B**). *PAX2* then regulates optic stalk development, while *PAX6* continues to define the eye fields (**B**). As development proceeds, fibroblast growth factors (FGFs) from surface ectoderm and transforming growth factor β (TGFβ) from surrounding mesenchyme stimulate optic cup development and formation of the inner (neural) and outer (pigmented) layers of the retina (**C**). *PAX6* is not necessary for optic cup formation. The transcription factors *MITF* and *CHX10* then direct further differentiation of these layers (**D**). *PAX6* expression in neural ectoderm in the eye fields at the neural plate stage also is essential for lens development. This expression upregulates *PAX6* and *SOX2* (another transcription factor) expression in prospective lens ectoderm. In turn, the optic stalk secretes BMP4, which maintains *SOX2* and initiates expression of another transcription factor *LMAF* in lens ectoderm (**E**). Together, *PAX6, SOX2,* and *LMAF* then regulate lens differentiation.

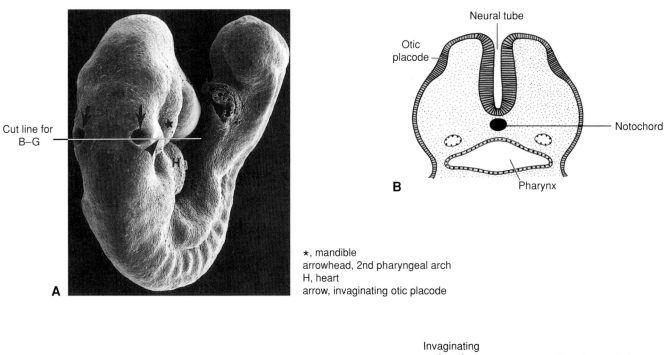

★, mandible
arrowhead, 2nd pharyngeal arch
H, heart
arrow, invaginating otic placode

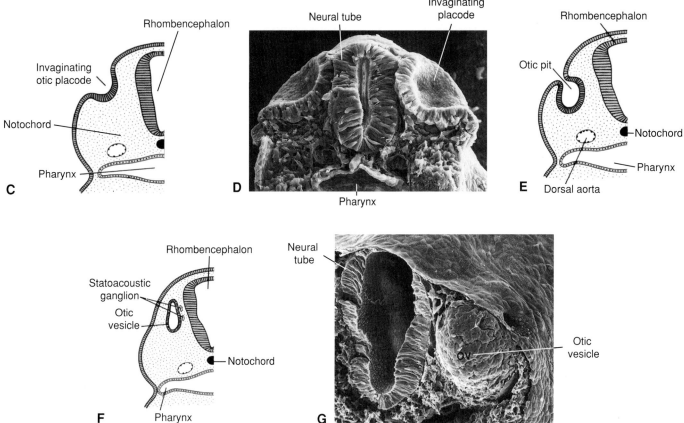

FIGURE 10.4. The ear consists of three different parts: the **external ear**, **middle ear**, and **internal ear**. The internal ear forms from **otic placodes (thickened ectoderm)** that develop on both sides of the hindbrain during the 4th week of development (**A** and **B**). These placodes invaginate to form otic vesicles (**C–G**).   (continued)

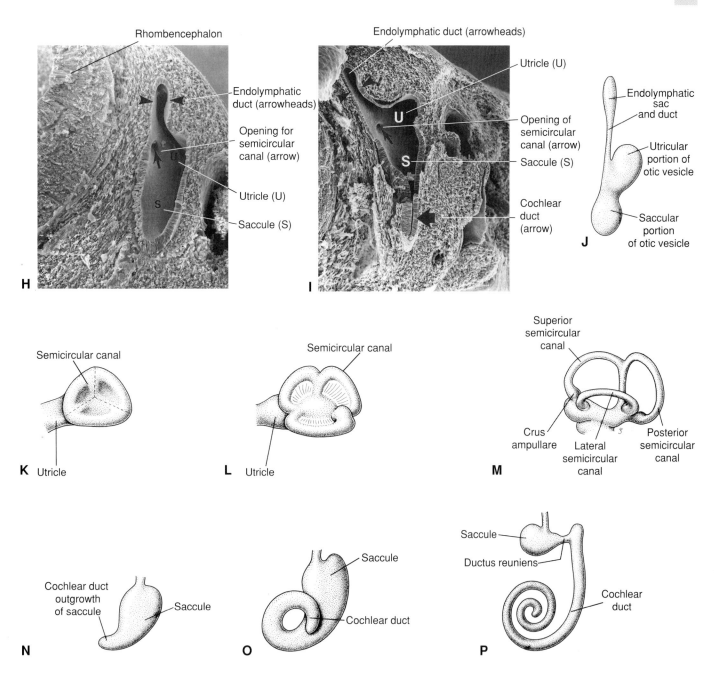

FIGURE 10.4. (*Continued*) The dorsal part of each otic vesicle forms an expansion called the **utricle**, from which the **endolymphatic duct** and **semicircular canals** grow (**H–M**). One end of each semicircular canal expands to form a **crus ampullare**, while the other end fails to widen (**M**). Cells in each crus ampullare then form a crest, called the **crista ampullare**, that contains sensory cells for maintenance of equilibrium. Similar sensory areas, called **maculae acousticae**, develop in the walls of the utricle. Changes in body position, detected by all of these sensory areas, are carried by **vestibular fibers** of the **vestibulocochlear nerve** (CN VIII). Dorsally, the vesicle also expands to form the **saccule** from which the **cochlear duct (organ of hearing)** grows (**H–J** and **N–P**). The connection between these two parts is called the **ductus reuniens** (**L**). Like the utricle, the saccule contains maculae acousticae for sensing changes in body position. Together, the saccule, utricle, semicircular canals, endolymphatic duct, and cochlea constitute the **membranous labyrinth** that becomes encased in bone (derived from surrounding mesenchyme) and forms the **bony labyrinth**.

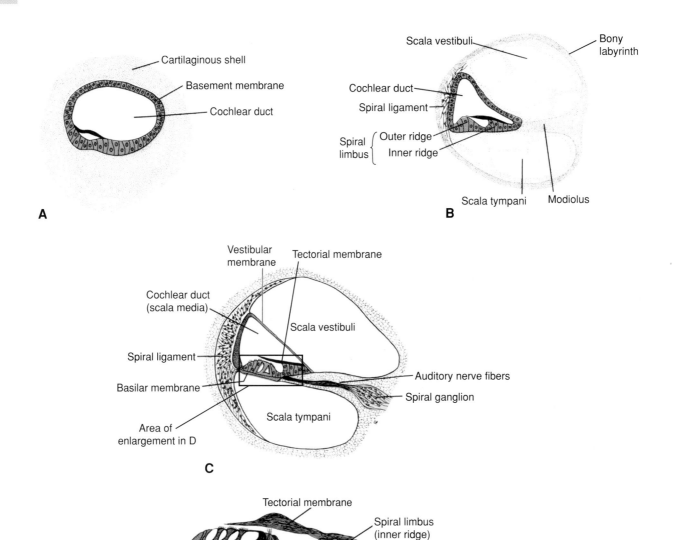

FIGURE 10.5. The **cochlear duct** lies between two fluid-filled chambers in the bony labyrinth, the **scala tympani** and the **scala vestibuli** (A–C). It is separated from the **scala vestibuli** by the **vestibular membrane** and from the **scala tympani** by the **basilar membrane** (C). In the 10th week, rows of **sensory hair cells** develop in the tissue of the cochlear duct that rests on the basilar membrane. Together the hair cells and overlying **tectorial membrane** constitute the **organ of Corti** (C and D). Hair cells are the sensory cells for hearing and, as the basilar membrane vibrates in the fluid filled membranous labyrinth, hair cells move against the tectorial membrane and are stimulated. Impulses generated by the hair cells are carried to the **spiral ganglion** on the inner side of the cochlear duct (C and D) and from there to the brain by **auditory fibers** of the **vestibulocochlear nerve** (CN VIII).

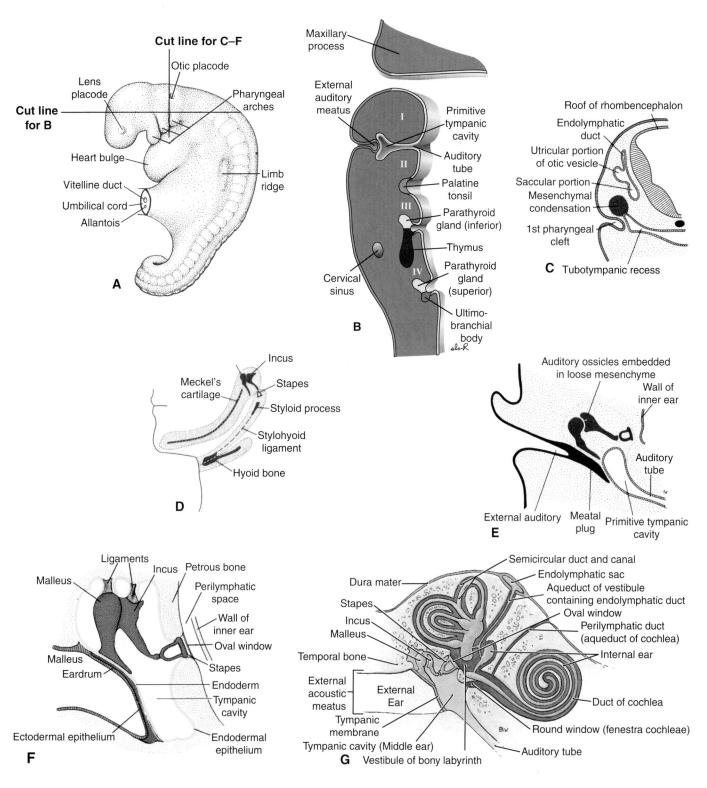

FIGURE 10.6. The **middle ear cavity** develops from the **tubotympanic recess** that forms as an extension of the 1st pharyngeal pouch (**A–C**; see Fig. 8.2). The **tympanic cavity** forms from an expansion of the distal part of this recess, while the proximal part of this pouch forms the **auditory tube**. Meanwhile the three **ear ossicles** develop from mesenchyme in the 1st (**malleus and incus**) and 2nd (**stapes**) pharyngeal arches (**D and E**). The **external auditory meatus** forms from the 1st pharyngeal cleft, and the **eardrum (tympanic membrane)** forms from the thin membrane separating the 1st cleft from the 1st pouch (**A–C**, **E and F**; see Fig. 8.2). Thus, the eardrum is covered by ectoderm on the outside and endoderm on the inside (**F**). In the 9th month, the malleus attaches to the **eardrum** and the stapes attaches to the **oval window**, a membrane-covered opening in the membranous labyrinth (**F and G**). Hearing occurs when sound causes vibrations in the eardrum that are transmitted from the malleus to the incus to the stapes to the oval window. These vibrations are then transmitted to the fluid-filled membranous labyrinth and from there to the organ of Corti, where hair cells are stimulated (**G**).

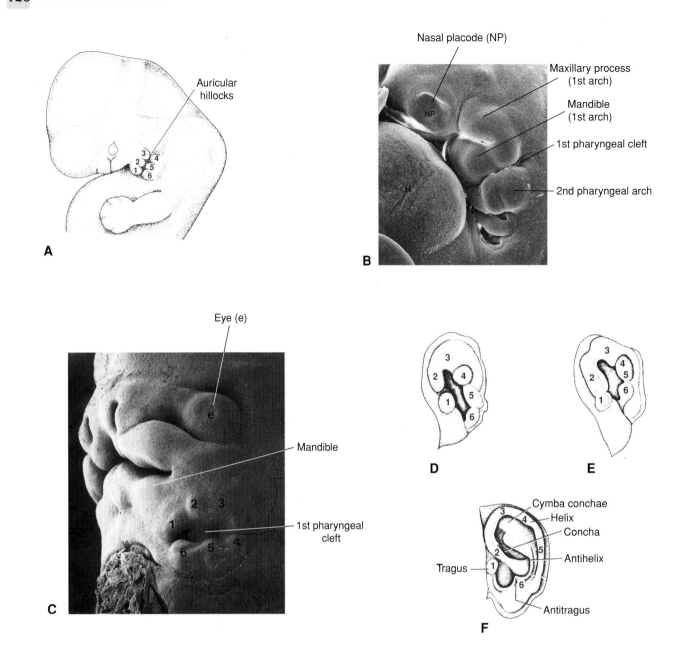

FIGURE 10.7. The **external ear** forms from the 1st and 2nd pharyngeal arches, which flank the 1st pharyngeal cleft (external auditory meatus; **A** and **B**). First, three **auricular hillocks** (swellings) on each arch appear as a result of proliferation of underlying mesenchyme (**A–C**). Eventually, through fusion and merging, these hillocks form the parts of the external ear (**D–F**). Interestingly, the ears begin development in almost a horizontal position at the back of the mandible (**C**). Then, as the mandible grows, the ears assume a more vertical and higher position on the side of the head. Sometimes the ears fail to achieve this location and remain in a low-set position. (continued)

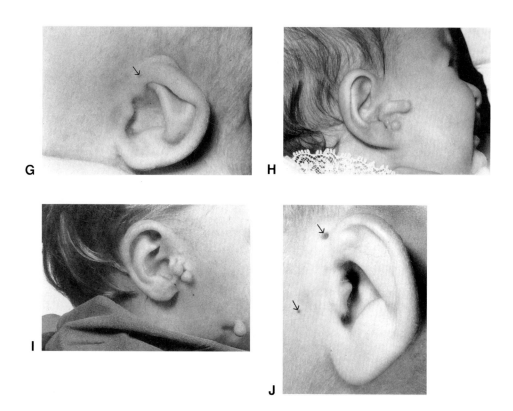

FIGURE 10.7. (*Continued*) Because of the complexity of ear development, birth defects involving these structures are common. Congenital deafness may result from abnormalities in the bony or membranous labyrinths or the ear ossicles and eardrum. Most cases are caused by genetic factors, but viruses (e.g., rubella virus) and chemical teratogens (e.g., retinoids) also can cause hearing loss. Gross defects of the external ear (**G**), or the presence of skin tags from formation of ectopic hillocks (**H** and **I**), or the presence of preauricular pits (**G** and **J**) are common and often are associated with malformations in other organ systems. In fact, all of the common syndromes, and most of the less common ones, include external ear anomalies as one of their defining characteristics. Therefore, any external ear defect indicates the need for a careful examination of the infant to rule out other birth defects.

CHAPTER 11

Fetal Period, Birth, and Birth Defects

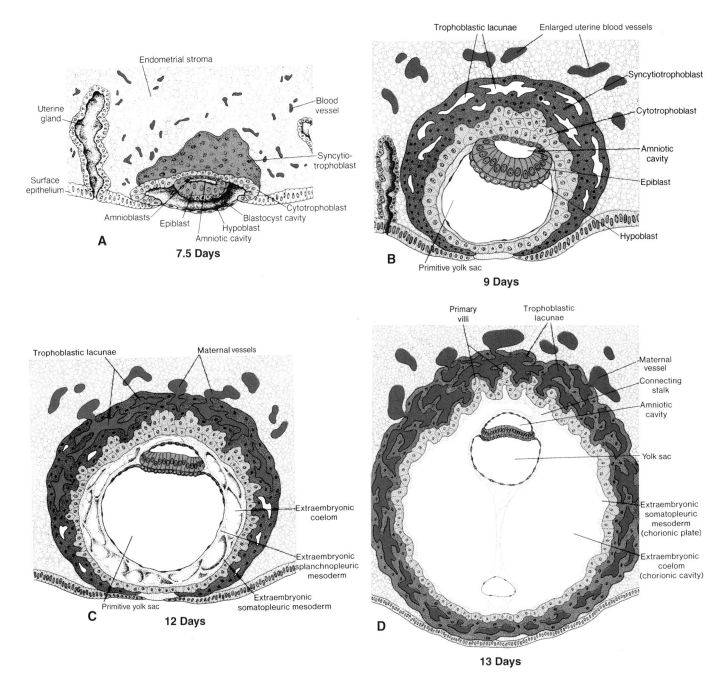

FIGURE 11.1.   Placental development begins 1 week after fertilization, when implantation is initiated, and involves the syncytiotrophoblast, cytotrophoblast, extraembryonic mesoderm, and uterine (endometrial layer) tissues (see Figs. 2.1 and 2.2). Shortly after the blastocyst contacts the uterine wall, the **syncytiotrophoblast** invades and erodes maternal tissues (**A**). By 9 days, it forms spaces within itself called **lacunae** (**lakes**; **B**). By 12 days, these "lakes" fill with maternal blood as the syncytiotrophoblast erodes uterine blood vessels (**C**). **Placental villi** begin to form by 13 days. These are **primary villi** that consist of a covering of syncytiotrophoblast and a core of **cytotrophoblast** and protrude into the lacunae (**D** and **E**).

(continued)

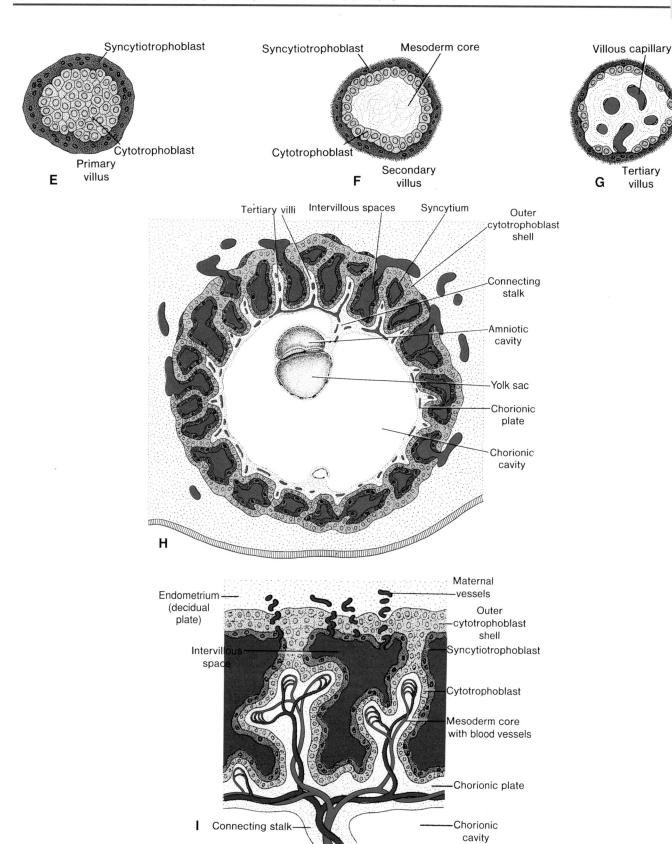

FIGURE 11.1. (*Continued*) Over the next several days, primary villi are invaded by **extraembryonic mesoderm** and become **secondary villi** (**E** and **F**). Blood vessels form in this extraembryonic mesoderm, in the **connecting stalk**, and in the embryo. The presence of these vessels creates **tertiary (definitive) villi** (**G** and **H**). Meanwhile, the cytotrophoblast grows through the syncytiotrophoblast and then connects with neighboring villi to form the outer cytotrophoblastic shell (**H**). Villi now extend from the **chorionic plate** (extraembryonic mesoderm) to the outer shell, and this shell anchors the placenta to the uterus along the **decidual plate** (**H** and **I**). Each villus consists of a mesodermal core, which contains blood vessels, covered by a layer of cytotrophoblast and a layer of syncytiotrophoblast (**I**).

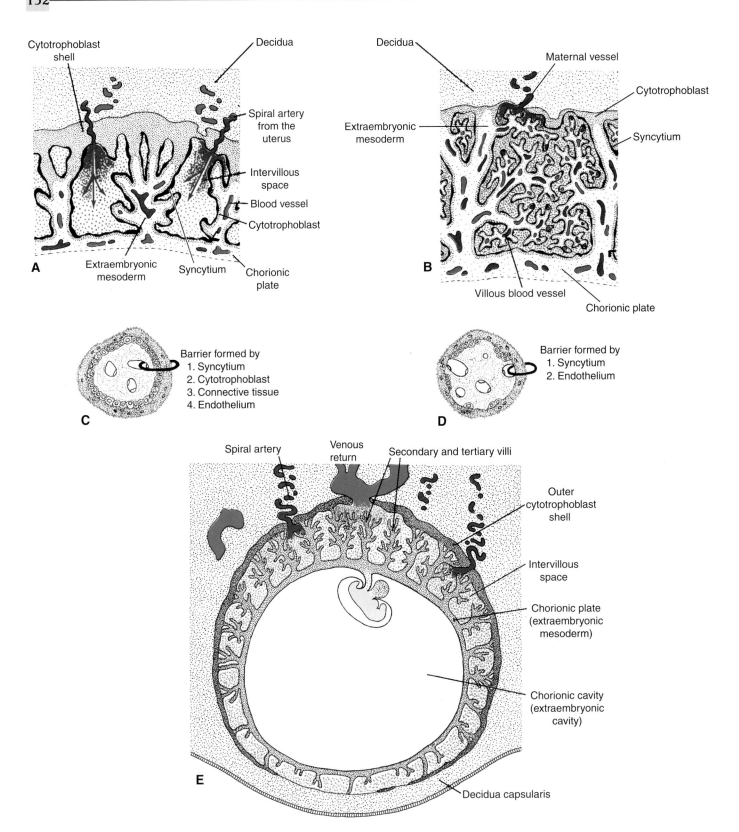

FIGURE 11.2. At the beginning of the 2nd month, as the heart develops, circulation in the placenta is established. Over the next several months, cytotrophoblast cells in the villi degenerate, leaving only a layer of syncytium between maternal blood on the outside and villus vessels on the inside (**A–D**). This thinning of villus walls facilitates diffusion across the membranes. Also in the 2nd month, villi on the abembryonic pole of the placenta degenerate (**E**), while those on the embryonic pole continue to grow and differentiate, creating the **chorionic frondosum (leafy chorion; E** and **F**). (continued)

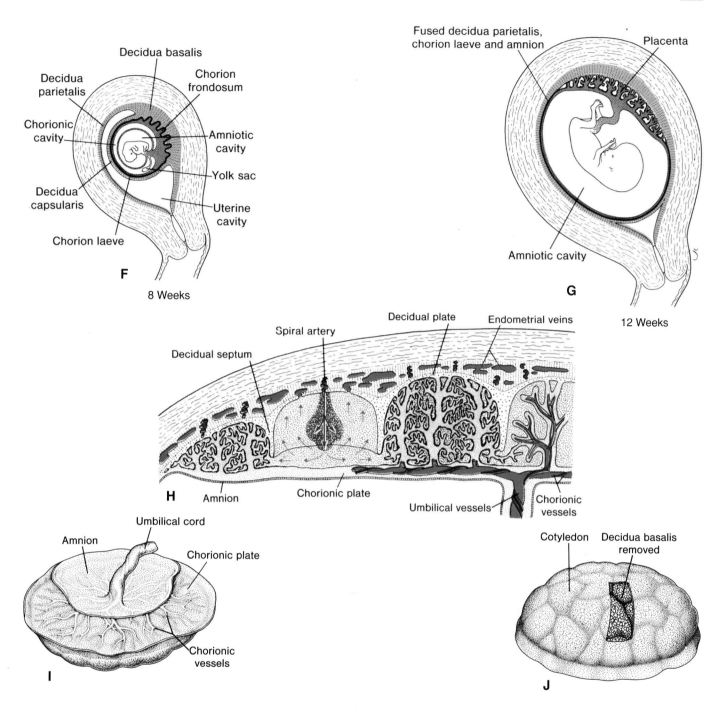

FIGURE 11.2. (*Continued*) Due to degeneration of villi, the abembryonic pole becomes smooth and forms the **chorion laeve** (**F**). At the same time, changes occur in the decidual layer of the endometrium lining the uterus. Thus, the decidua over the chorionic frondosum forms the **decidua basalis**, which consists of a layer of large cells that form the **decidual plate** (**F**). These cells are tightly adherent to the cytotrophoblastic shell and anchor the placenta. The decidual layer over the abembryonic pole forms the **decidua capsularis**, while decidua over the remainder of the uterus forms the **decidua parietalis** (**F**) By the end of the 3rd month, as the baby grows, the decidua capsularis contacts the decidua parietalis on the opposite wall of the uterus and breaks down so that the chorion fuses with this wall (**F** and **G**). Then, as the amniotic cavity expands and fills with additional fluid, the amnion contacts the chorionic laeve and the chorionic cavity is obliterated (**G**). Meanwhile, in the 4th and 5th months, septa from the decidual plate grow down to separate clusters of villi into compartments called **cotyledons** (**H**). These septa do not grow down sufficiently to contact the chorionic plate, so maternal blood can flow between the cotyledons that form (**H**). Maternal blood is delivered to the cotyledons by **spiral arteries**. The blood then circulates around the villi and is returned to the maternal system by **endometrial veins**. Because villi branch extensively to create tree-like structures with a great amount of surface area, the exchange of nutrients and metabolic and gaseous products is enhanced, although there is no mixing of maternal and fetal blood (**H**). In addition to performing these exchanges, the placenta produces **progesterone** and **estrogenic hormones**, human chorionic gonadotropin (hCG; used for pregnancy tests), and somatomammotropin, a growth hormone that gives the fetus priority on nutrients in maternal blood. At term the placenta is discoid, with a diameter of 15 to 20 cm, weighs about 500 to 600 g, and is "delivered" approximately 30 minutes after birth of the baby (**I** and **J**).

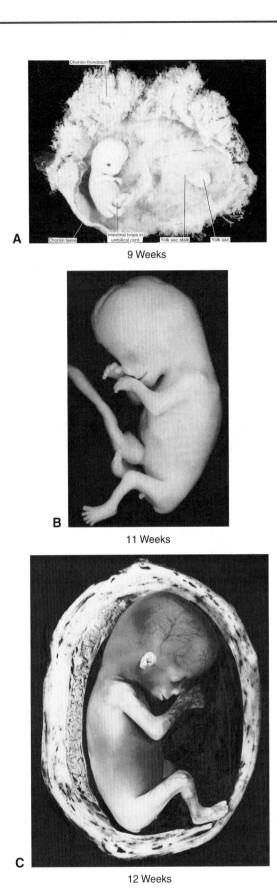

A 9 Weeks

B 11 Weeks

C 12 Weeks

FIGURE 11.3. The **fetal period** of development begins in the 9th week (**A**). By this time, all of the organ primordia have been established and are growing and continuing their differentiation. From the 3rd to the 5th months, the fetus lengthens rapidly (**A–E**), and its age can be estimated by measuring the **crown–rump length (CRL)**, from the top of the head to the buttocks (Table 11.1). Weight gain occurs mostly in the last 3 months, when 50% of the full-term weight is added (Table 11.1). Respiratory movements start in the 3rd to 4th months, and general movements of the fetus can be detected by the mother in the 5th month. Some sounds can be heard by the fetus in the 6th month, and the eyes become sensitive to light in the 7th month (Table 11.2).   (continued)

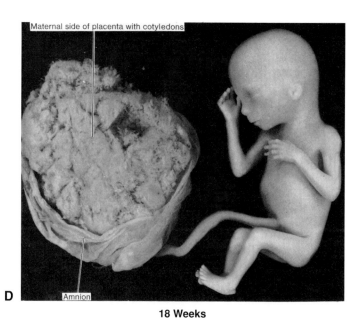

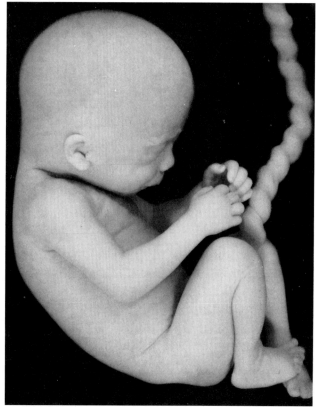

D Maternal side of placenta with cotyledons — Amnion

18 Weeks

E **7 Months**

Table 11.1. **Growth in Length and Weight During the Fetal Period**

Gestational Age (wk)	CRL (cm)	Weight (g)
9–12	5–8	10–45
13–16	9–14	60–200
17–20	15–19	250–450
21–24	20–23	500–820
25–28	24–27	900–1300
29–32	28–30	1400–2100
33–36	31–34	2200–2900
37–38	35–36	3000–3400

CRL, crown–rump length.

Table 11.2. **Developmental Horizons During Fetal Life**

Event	Gestational Age (wk)
Taste buds appear	7
Swallowing	10
Respiratory movements	14–16
Sucking movements	24
Some sounds can be heard	24–26
Eyes sensitive to light*	28

*Recognition of form and color occurs postnatally.

FIGURE 11.3. *(Continued)* The normal gestation period is **40 weeks** after the **last normal menstrual period (LNMP)** or, more accurately, **38 weeks after fertilization**. During the last 2 weeks, the uterus undergoes a transitional phase in preparation for **birth (parturition)**, including a thickening of the myometrium (muscle layer) in the upper region of the uterus and a thinning in the lower region and cervix. The signals that initiate **labor** have not yet been determined, but the labor process itself has three stages. The first of these is **effacement** (thinning and shortening) and **dilation of the cervix**. This stage is produced by uterine contractions that force the amniotic sac against the cervical canal like a wedge, or, if the membranes have ruptured, the fetal head exerts the pressure. The second stage is **delivery of the fetus**, which is assisted by uterine contractions, but is accomplished primarily by increasing intra-abdominal pressure through abdominal muscle contractions. The third, and final, stage of labor is **delivery of the placenta and fetal membranes**, which is accomplished by uterine and abdominal wall contractions. Uterine contractions are directional, going from top to bottom, and usually begin at 10-minute intervals. During the second stage of labor, contractions occur less than 1 minute apart and last from 60 to 90 seconds each.

Dizygotic Twinning

Monozygotic Twinning

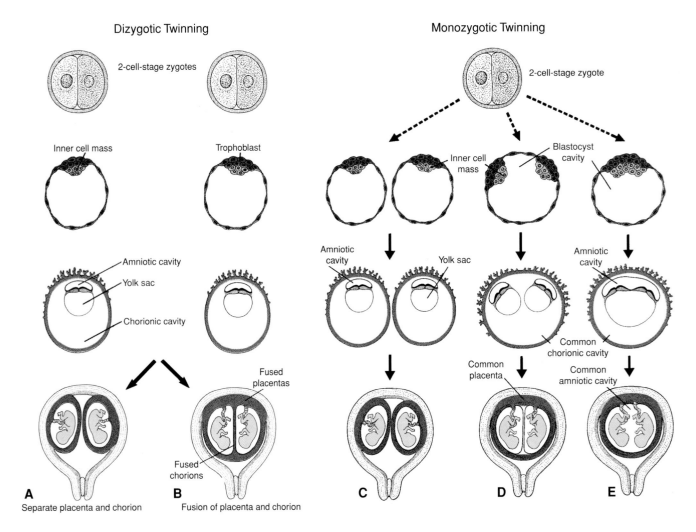

A Separate placenta and chorion

B Fusion of placenta and chorion

FIGURE 11.4. Some infants are born **prematurely** (preterm infants; less than 34 weeks gestation) and are subject to increased morbidity and mortality. In fact, prematurity is a leading cause of infant mortality, accounting for approximately 25 % of all infant deaths. Unfortunately, the incidence of premature births is increasing, in part because of multiple conception pregnancies (e.g., twins, triplets) due to the increased use of fertility drugs. Approximately 12 % of preterm infants are **twins**, who often are of low birth weight. About two thirds of twins are **dizygotic** (derived from separate fertilized eggs), occurring with a frequency of 7 to 11 per 1000 births (**A** and **B**); the other one third are **monozygotic**, occurring in 3 to 4 per 1000 births (**C–E**). In monozygotic twins, the earliest separation occurs at the two-cell stage (**C**). Usually, however, splitting of the zygote occurs at the early blastocyst stage with division of the inner cell mass, leaving the two embryos with a common placenta and common chorionic cavities, but with separate amnionic cavities (**D**). In rare instances, the split may occur at the bilaminar disc stage, leaving two embryos with a common amnion and chorion and a single placenta (**E**).   (continued)

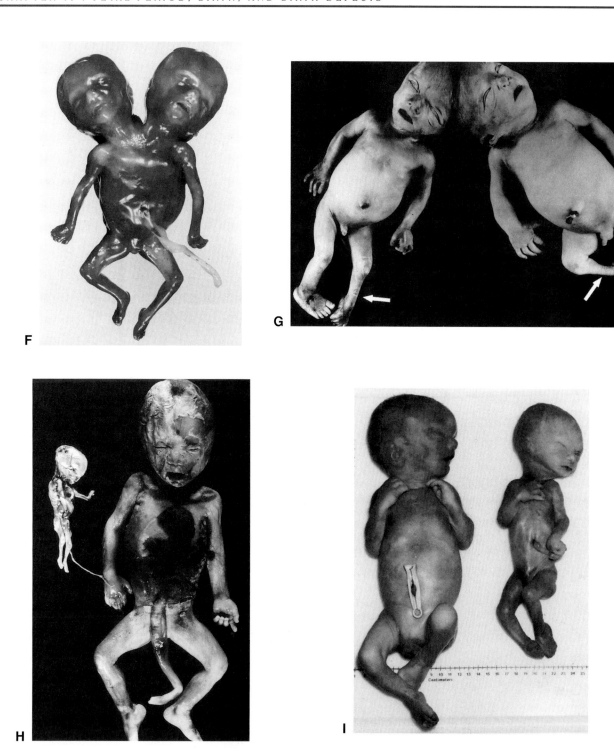

FIGURE 11.4. (*Continued*) Sometimes, separation of the inner cell mass or germ disc may be incomplete, resulting in **conjoined (Siamese) twins** (**F** and **G**). These twins also may arise by fusion of two germ discs. Twinning is an anomaly, and only about 29% of twins that are conceived are born alive. Of these, 10% to 20% die, compared to 2% of infants from single pregnancies. Occasionally, one twin is incompletely resorbed, resulting in a **fetus papyraceus** (**H**). In other cases, one twin receives most of the placental blood flow due to anastomoses between placental vessels, a condition called **twin transfusion syndrome** (**I**). In these situations, one twin is larger than the other, and in 60% to 100% of cases, both twins die.

Risk of Birth Defects Being Induced

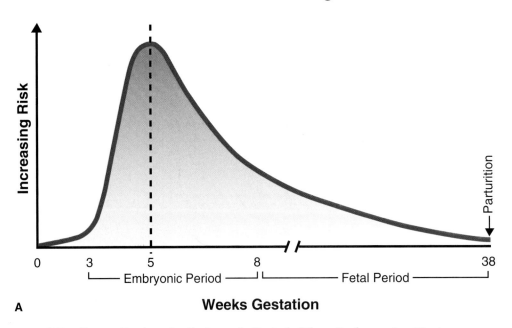

A

Weeks Gestation

Table 11.3. **Summary of Key Events During the Embryonic Period. When Embryos Are Most Sensitive to Teratogenic Insult**

Days	Somites	Length (cm)	Characteristic Features
14–15	0	0.2	Appearance of primitive streak
16–18	0	0.4	Notochordal process appears; hematopoietic cells in yolk sac
19–20	0	1.0–2.0	Intraembryonic mesoderm spread under cranial ectoderm; primitive streak continues; umbilical vessels and cranial folds beginning to form
20–21	1–4	2.0–3.0	Cranial neural folds elevated and deep neural groove established; embryo beginning to bend
22–33	5–12	3.0–3.5	Fusion of neural folds begins in cervical region; cranial and caudal neuropores open widely; 1st and 2nd visceral arches present; heart tube beginning to fold
24–25	13–20	3.0–4.5	Cephalocaudal folding under way; cranial neuropore closing or closed; optic vesicles formed; otic placodes appear
26–27	21–29	3.5–5.0	Caudal neuropore closing or closed; upper limb buds appear; three pairs of visceral arches
28–30	30–35	4.0–6.0	Fourth visceral arch formed; hindlimb buds appear; otic vesicle and lens placode form
31–35		7.0–10.0	Forelimbs paddle-shaped; nasal pits formed; embryo tightly C-shaped
36–42		9.0–14.0	Digital rays in hand and footplates; brain vesicles prominent; external auricle forming from auricular hillocks; umbilical herniation initiated
43–49		13.0–22.0	Pigmentation of retina visible; digital rays separating; nipples and eyelids formed; maxillary swellings fuse with medial nasal swellings as upper lip forms; prominent umbilical herniation
50–56		21.0–31.0	Limbs long, bent at elbows, knees; fingers, toes free; face more human-like; tail disappears; umbilical herniation persists to end of 3rd month

FIGURE 11.5. **Birth defect, congenital malformation,** and **congenital anomaly** are synonymous terms used to describe structural, behavioral, and metabolic disorders present at birth. **Teratology** is the science that studies the origin and causes of birth defects. Birth defects are common, with major structural anomalies occurring in 4% to 6% of all infants. Like prematurity, they are a leading cause of infant mortality, accounting for approximately 25% of infant deaths. They are also costly in terms of emotional trauma for the affected child and his or her family, hospital expenses, and health insurance. Yet, many birth defects are preventable. Seventy percent of **neural tube defects** (e.g., **spina bifida** and **anencephaly**; see Fig. 3.10) could be prevented through maternal use of supplemental **folic acid** (400 µg) taken daily beginning 2 to 3 months prior to conception and continuing throughout gestation. All defects caused by maternal diabetes can be prevented if prospective mothers are placed on strict metabolic control of their disease prior to conception. All defects caused by maternal ingestion of alcohol and other drugs can be prevented if the mother stops use of the substance prior to conception and throughout pregnancy. All defects caused by iodine and vitamin deficiencies could be avoided by supplements containing these missing nutrients. Many defects caused by exposure to environmental and pharmaceutical compounds could be avoided by eliminating the mother's exposure, e.g., by avoiding placing women of childbearing age in positions that require exposure to such potential environmental dangers in the workplace or postponing dental x-rays, or by having the physician prescribe a less damaging drug. The most important issue for successful prevention strategies is initiating them prior to conception, because most malformations are caused early in gestation (during the 2nd to 8th weeks), when women often do not realize they are pregnant (**A**). This is the period of organogenesis, when organ systems are just beginning to form (Table 11.3), and cells that are rapidly proliferating, migrating, and differentiating are most susceptible to insult. Defects also may arise later in gestation, so no part of pregnancy is entirely safe from the effects of teratogens. (continued)

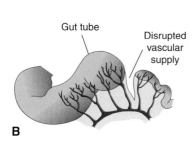

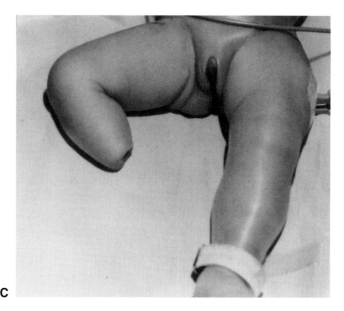

Table 11.4. **Teratogens Associated With Human Malformations**

Teratogen	Congential Malformations
Infectious agent	
Rubella virus	Cataracts, glaucoma, heart defects, deafness, tooth defects
Cytomegalovirus	Microcephaly, blindness, mental retardation, fetal death
Herpes simplex virus	Microphthalmia, microcephaly, retinal dysplasia
Varicella virus	Limb hypoplasia, mental retardation, muscle atrophy
Human immunodeficiency virus	Microcephaly, growth retardation
Toxoplasmosis	Hydrocephalus, cerebral calcifications, microphthalmia
Syphilis	Mental retardation, deafness
Physical agents	
X-rays	Microcephaly, spina bifida, cleft palate, limb defects
Hyperthermia	Anencephaly, spina bifida, mental retardation, facial defects
Obesity	Neural tube defects
Chemical agents	
Thalidomide	Limb defects, heart malformations
Aminopterin	Anencephaly, hydrocephaly, cleft lip and palate
Diphenylhydantoin (phenytoin)	Fetal hydantoin syndrome: facial defects, mental retardation
Valproic acid	Neural tube defects; heart, craniofacial, and limb anomalies
Trimethadione	Cleft palate, heart defects, urogenital and skeletal abnormalities
Lithium	Heart malformations
Amphetamines	Cleft lip and palate, heart defects
Warfarin	Chondrodysplasia, microcephaly
Angiotensin-converting enzyme (ACE) inhibitors	Growth retardation, fetal death
Cocaine	Growth retardation, microcephaly, behavioral abnormalities, gastroschisis
Alcohol	Fetal alcohol syndrome, short palpebral fissures, maxillary hypoplasia, heart defects, mental retardation
Isotretinoin (vitamin A)	Vitamin A embryopathy: small, abnormally shaped ears; mandibular hypoplasia; cleft palate; heart defects
Industrial solvents	Low birth weight, craniofacial and neural tube defects
Organic mercury	Neurologic symptoms similar to those of cerebral palsy
Lead	Growth retardation, neurologic disorders
Hormones	
Androgenic agents (e.g., ethisterone, norethisterone)	Masculinization of female genitalia; fused labia, clitoral hypertrophy
Diethylstilbestrol (DES)	Malformation of the uterus, uterine tubes, and upper vagina; vaginal cancer; malformed testes
Endocrine disruptors (environmental estrogens)	Reduced sperm counts; hypospadias; reproductive tract abnormalities
Maternal diabetes	Variety of malformations; heart and neural tube defects most common

FIGURE 11.5. (*Continued*) Sometimes defects arise after structures have already formed. For example, **disruptions** occur when a structure that has developed normally becomes altered due to destructive forces, such as **"vascular accidents"** that cause bowel atresias (**B**; see Fig. 6.7C–F) or amniotic bands that cause limb or digit amputations (**C**; see Fig. 4.8E). Deformations also occur later in pregnancy due to mechanical forces, such as when a uterine cavity is too small and the baby develops clubbed feet. Causes for birth defects include genetic factors (15 %); environmental factors (10 %; Table 11.4); a combination of genetic and environmental factors (multifactorial causes; 25 %); and twinning (0.5–1 %). However, in most cases the cause is unknown (40–60 %). Sometimes a group of defects occur together and the specific cause is known. These cases are designated **syndromes**, such as Down syndrome (trisomy 21), caused by an extra chromosome 21, and fetal alcohol syndrome (FAS), caused by maternal alcohol abuse.

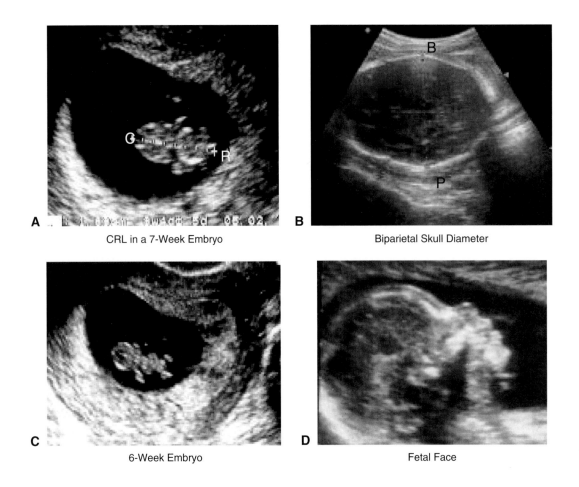

A — CRL in a 7-Week Embryo

B — Biparietal Skull Diameter

C — 6-Week Embryo

D — Fetal Face

FIGURE 11.6. **Prenatal diagnosis** techniques have made it possible to identify birth defects prior to delivery and are resulting in better care at the time of birth as well as development of fetal surgical techniques to correct some abnormalities in utero (e.g., diaphragmatic hernias, spina bifida). **Prenatal ultrasound** is a popular noninvasive technique that can estimate fetal age by measuring crown–rump length (**A**), biparietal diameter (**B**) and circumference of the head, and can determine the degree of ossification in various regions. Resolution of the images obtained has improved greatly as newer techniques and approaches have been developed (**C** and **D**). (continued)

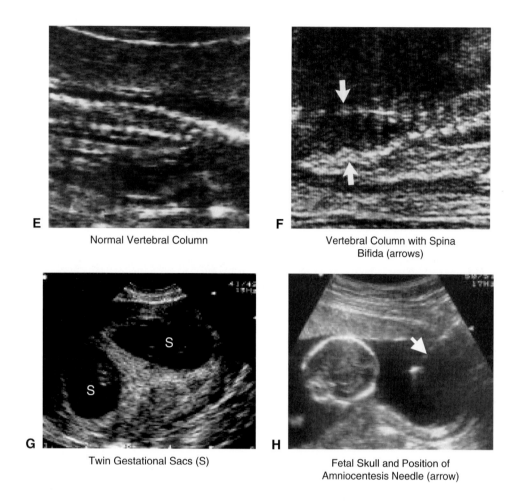

E Normal Vertebral Column

F Vertebral Column with Spina
Bifida (arrows)

G Twin Gestational Sacs (S)

H Fetal Skull and Position of
Amniocentesis Needle (arrow)

FIGURE 11.6.   (*Continued*) Ultrasound also can be used to identify many potential problems, including the presence of birth defects, such as spina bifida (**E** and **F**), and twins (**G**). **Amniocentesis** is a technique in which a needle is placed through the mother's abdomen and the placenta into the amniotic cavity (**H**). Fluid is obtained and analyzed for the presence of proteins, chemicals, and electrolytes that offer insights into fetal health. For example, **alpha-fetoprotein (AFP)** is elevated in cases of neural tube defects. This protein also is elevated in maternal blood in such cases and can be detected through maternal serum screening. Fetal cells floating in amniotic fluid samples can be collected, grown in culture, and analyzed for chromosomal abnormalities. Chorionic villus biopsy (CVS) is another technique used to obtain cells. In this procedure a needle is inserted into the placenta and villus cells are withdrawn. These cells can then be analyzed for genetic anomalies.

GLOSSARY OF KEY TERMS

Adenohypophysis Anterior portion of the pituitary derived from Rathke's pouch

Alar plates Sensory area in the dorsal region of the spinal cord and brain

Allantois Vestigial structure that serves as a respiratory organ for avian embryos. It extends from the ventral region of the urogenital sinus to the umbilicus. Later, its distal portion, the urachus, becomes a fibrous cord and forms the median umbilical ligament. If it remains patent, it may form a urachal fistula or cyst in this region.

Alveolar cells Cells lining the alveoli. Type I cells are involved in gas exchange; type II cells produce surfactant.

Amnion Membrane derived from the epiblast that surrounds the fluid-filled amniotic cavity around the embryo and fetus. The fluid cushions the fetus and forms a hydrostatic wedge to assist with dilation of the cervix during labor. The fluid itself can be used for analysis of fetal well-being.

Amniocentesis Procedure used to withdraw amniotic fluid for analysis of factors such as alpha-fetoprotein (AFP) and cells (chromosomes) that provide information about the status of the fetus

Anencephaly Neural tube defect in which the cranial neural folds fail to close, leading to tissue degeneration and little or no formation of higher brain centers, cerebral cortex, and other neurologic structures. The abnormality is lethal, but 70% of these defects can be prevented by daily maternal consumption of 400 μg of folic acid beginning 2 to 3 months prior to conception and continuing throughout pregnancy.

Annulus fibrosis Outer ring of fibrous tissue in an intervertebral disc

Antimüllerian hormone Another term for the müllerian-inhibiting substance produced by Sertoli cells that causes regression of the müllerian (paramesonephric) ducts in males

Aortic arch Branch from the aortic sac to the dorsal aorta traveling in the center of each pharyngeal arch. Initially, there are five pairs, but these undergo considerable remodeling to form definitive vascular patterns for the head and neck, aorta, and pulmonary circulation.

Apical ectodermal ridge (AER) Layer of thickened ectoderm at the distal tip of the limb that controls outgrowth of the limb by maintaining a rapidly proliferating population of adjacent mesoderm cells, that form the progress zone

Apoptosis Programmed cell death, e.g., between the digits

Atresia Congenital absence of an opening or lumen, e.g., gut atresia

Autonomic nervous system The sympathetic and parasympathetic nervous systems that control smooth muscle and glands

Basal plates Motor area in the ventral portion of the spinal cord and brain

Bone morphogenetic proteins (BMPs) Members of the transforming growth factor β family that serve as signal molecules for a number of morphogenetic events, e.g., including dorsalizing the CNS, participating in bone formation

Bowman's capsule Cup-shaped structure at the end of each proximal convoluted tubule that partially surrounds a glomerulus

Brainstem "Lower" centers of the brain, including the myelencephalon, pons of the metencephalon, and the mesencephalon

Buccopharyngeal membrane Membrane formed at the cranial end of the germ disc by adhesion between epiblast and hypoblast cells. Later, it covers the opening of the oral cavity and breaks down as the pharynx develops.

Cardinal veins System of anterior, posterior, and common cardinal veins that drain the head and body of the embryo in the late 3rd and early 4th weeks

Cerebral aqueduct (of Sylvius) Lumen of the mesencephalon that connects the 3rd and 4th ventricles. It often is the site for abnormalities that impede the flow of cerebrospinal fluid and cause hydrocephalus.

Chondrocranium Part of the neurocranium that forms the base of the skull that arises by first establishing cartilage models for the bones (endochondral ossification)

Chorion Multilayered structure consisting of the somatic layer of extraembryonic mesoderm, cytotrophoblast, and syncytiotrophoblast. It contributes the fetal portion of the placenta, including the villi and villus lakes.

Chorion frondosum (leafy chorion) Embryonic side of the chorion, where villi form

Chorion laeve (smooth chorion) Abembryonic side of the chorion, where villi regress, leaving a smooth surface

Choroid plexuses Vascularized structures formed in the lateral, 3rd, and 4th ventricles that produce cerebrospinal fluid

Cloaca Common chamber for the hindgut and urinary systems. Its anterior portion forms the urogenital sinus, and its posterior portion forms the anus.

Cloacal membrane (plate) Membrane formed at the caudal end of the embryo from adhesion between epiblast and hypoblast cells. Later, it covers the cloaca and eventually breaks down to form openings into the urogenital sinus and anus.

Coloboma Defect in the eye due to incomplete closure of the optic fissure. These defects usually are restricted to the iris.

Compaction Process whereby cells of the morula stage form tight junctions to seal themselves in preparation for forming and pumping fluid into the blastocyst cavity

Congenital malformation Synonymous with the term birth defect; refers to any structural, behavioral, functional, or metabolic disorder present at birth

Cranial nerves (CN) 12 pairs of nerves associated with the brain, all but two of which (the olfactory and optic) originate from the brainstem

Craniosynostosis Premature closure of one or more cranial sutures leading to abnormally shaped skulls. A major cause are mutations in fibroblast growth factor receptors (FGFRs).

Cryptorchidism Failure of one or both testes to descend to the scrotum

Cytotrophoblast Proliferative inner layer of the trophoblast

Deformations Altered development of structures caused by mechanical forces, e.g., clubbed feet resulting from too little room in the amniotic cavity.

Dermatome The dorsal portion of each somite that forms the dermis of the skin. Dermatomes are segmented and are supplied by spinal nerves from the segments at which they originated. This segmental pattern is maintained as the dermatomes migrate over the body. Thus, each region that they occupy on the skin also is called a dermatome and is innervated by the same spinal nerve that originally supplied the dermatome region of the somite.

Diaphysis Shaft of the long bones

Diencephalon Derived from the caudal portion of the prosencephalon (forebrain); forms the thalamus, hypothalamus, posterior lobe of the pituitary, optic stalks (nerves), and other structures

Dihydrotestosterone Converted from testosterone and responsible for differentiation of the mesonephric duct and external genitalia

Disruptions Term used to describe birth defects resulting from destructive processes that alter a structure that initially had formed normally, e.g., vascular accidents that cause bowel atresias, and amniotic bands that cause limb or digit amputations

Dizygotic twins Twins formed from two separate eggs; the most common form of twinning (66%)

Dorsal mesentery Double layer of peritoneum suspending the gut tube from the dorsal body wall from the lower end of the esophagus to the rectum. Later, as the gut grows and rotates, some parts of the dorsal mesentery are lost as portions of the gut fuse to the posterior body wall, e.g. parts of the duodenum and colon.

Dorsal primary ramus Branch of a spinal nerve that innervates muscles derived from the epimere and skin over the back

Dorsal root Sensory fibers passing from a dorsal root ganglion to the spinal cord

Ectoderm One of the three basic germ layers that forms skin, the central nervous system, hair, and many other structures

Ectopic Something that is not in its normal position, e.g., an embryo's implantation site

Efferent ductules Tubules that connect the rete testes to the mesonephric duct for the passage of sperm from the seminiferous tubules to the epididymis. The tubules are derived from nephric tubules of the mesonephric kidney.

Endocardial cushions Structures consisting of loose connective tissue covered by endothelium that are responsible for most septation processes occurring in the heart

Endoderm One of three basic germ layers that forms the gut and its derivatives

Endochondral ossification Mechanism for forming bone by first establishing a cartilaginous model followed by ossification. This type of bone formation is characteristic of the bones of the limbs and base of the skull.

Epiblast The dorsal (top) layer of cells that makes up the bilaminar germ disc during the 2nd week of development. The hypoblast forms the ventral layer. All tissues of the embryo are derived from the epiblast.

Epibranchial placodes Four thickened regions of ectoderm lying dorsal to the pharyngeal arches that form sensory ganglia for cranial nerves V, VII, IX, and X

Epididymis Highly convoluted tube derived from the mesonephric duct and used for sperm storage

Epimere Dorsal musculature derived from the myotome portion of each somite that forms the extensor muscles of the back

Epiphysis An end of one of the long bones

Epiphyseal plate Cartilaginous region between the diaphysis and epiphysis of the long bones that continues to produce bone growth by endochondral ossification until the bones have acquired their full length. Then these plates disappear (close).

Epiploic foramen (of Winslow) Opening between the lesser and greater sacs in the abdominal cavity located at the free margin of the lesser omentum between the duodenum and the liver. In its ventral border lie the common bile duct, hepatic artery, and portal vein (the portal triad).

Fibroblast growth factors (FGFs) Signal proteins in a large family having over 15 members. They are involved in a number of embryological events, including formation of the sutures and bones of the skull. Mutations in their receptors (FGFRs) cause a variety of craniofacial abnormalities, including many forms of craniosynostosis.

Fistula An abnormal passageway

Folic acid A B vitamin that can prevent approximately 70% of neural tube defects if taken as a 400 μg supplement by women beginning 2 to 3 months prior to conception and continuing throughout pregnancy

Foramen cecum Pit at the junction of the anterior two thirds and posterior one third of the tongue representing the site of origin of the thyroid gland

Foramen ovale Opening in the interatrial septum that permits shunting of blood from right to left during fetal development

Fossa ovalis Depression on the right side of the interatrial septum formed when the septum primum and septum secundum are pressed against each other and the foramen ovale is closed at birth

Foregut Part of the gut tube beginning caudal to the pharynx just proximal to the lung bud and extending to a point just distal to the liver bud. It forms the esophagus, stomach, and part of the duodenum in addition to the lungs, liver, gallbladder, and pancreas, all of which form from diverticula (buds) off the gut tube.

Gastrulation Process of forming the three primary germ layers from the epiblast involving movement of cells through the primitive streak to form endoderm and mesoderm

Germ layers Three basic cell layers of ectoderm, mesoderm, and endoderm derived from the process of gastrulation. These layers form all of the structures in the embryo.

Glomerulus Tuft of capillaries formed in Bowman's capsule at the end of each proximal convoluted tubule.

Gray rami communicantes Connections carrying postganglionic sympathetic fibers from ganglia in the sympathetic trunks to spinal nerves. Gray rami exist at all levels of the spinal cord.

Greater omentum Double layer of peritoneum formed from dorsal mesentery and extending down over the intestines from the greater curvature of the stomach. It serves as a storage site for fat and can wall off pockets of infection (the "policeman of the abdomen").

Greater sac Most of the abdominal cavity, with the exception of the lesser sac lying dorsal to the lesser omentum. The two sacs are connected via the epiploic foramen (of Winslow).

Growth factors Proteins that act as signal molecules; they usually are secreted and have their signals transduced by receptors on target cells.

Gubernaculum Condensation of mesenchyme extending from the testis to the floor of the scrotum that assists in descent of the testis from the posterior abdominal wall to the scrotum

Hindgut Part of the gut tube extending from the distal one third of the transverse colon to the upper portion of the anal canal. It forms part of the transverse colon, the descending colon, sigmoid colon, rectum, and upper part of the anal canal.

Homeobox genes Transcription factors that contain a homeobox, a specific DNA-binding motif (sequence) within a region called the homeodomain. These genes are important for patterning the embryonic axis, establishing different regions of the brain, determining the origin and type of gut derivatives, patterning the limbs, and other similar phenomena.

Hydrocephalus Increased amounts of cerebrospinal fluid in the brain, leading to increased intracranial pressure. Usually due to a block in the circulatory pattern of the fluid which most often occurs in the cerebral aqueduct of Sylvius in the mesencephalon. If the cranial sutures have not fused, the child's head enlarges, sometimes to great proportions if the pressure is not relieved.

Hypomere Musculature derived from the dorsolateral portion of each somite; forms muscles of the anterior body wall

Hypertrophy An increase in size of a part or organ

Hyperplasia An increase in cell number

Hypoblast Ventral layer of the bilaminar germ disc. It contributes to formation of the yolk sac and extraembryonic mesoderm, but not to tissues of the embryo.

Hypospadias An opening of the urethra along the ventral aspect of the penis or scrotum

Inguinal canal Oblique passageway from the lower abdomen to the scrotum for the testes; forms in females as well

Inner cell mass Cluster of cells segregated to one pole of the blastocyst and from which the entire embryo develops

Intermaxillary segment Formed from the medial nasal processes, it includes the philtrum region of the upper lip, the upper jaw component housing the four incisor teeth, and the primary palate.

Intermediate column Origin of the sympathetic cell bodies (lateral horn cells) in the spinal cord from T1 to L2

Intermediate mesoderm Mesoderm-derived layer lying between the paraxial and lateral plate layers and responsible for forming much of the urogenital system

Intervertebral disc Cushioning disc between each vertebra and the next; consists of a central gelatinous portion called the nucleus pulposus and an outer ring of fibrous tissue called the annulus fibrosus

Intraperitoneal Describes organs suspended in the abdominal cavity by a mesentery

Karyotype The chromosomal make-up of an individual

Lateral plate mesoderm Mesoderm-derived tissue that splits into the splanchnopleure (visceral) and somatopleure (somatic) layers surrounding the body cavity

Laterality The existence of right and left sides established during gastrulation in the 3rd week of development. Patients with defects in sidedness, such that they are primarily bilaterally right- or left-sided, have laterality sequences.

Lesser sac Space behind the lesser omentum that communicates with the rest of the abdominal cavity (greater sac) via the epiploic foramen (of Winslow)

Lesser omentum Double layer of peritoneum forming part of the ventral mesentery and extending from the liver to the proximal end of the

duodenum and lesser curvature of the stomach

Mantle layer Inner layer of the neural tube containing neurons (gray matter)

Marginal layer Peripheral layer of the neural tube containing nerve fibers (white matter)

Membranous ossification Process of forming bone directly from mesenchyme. This process is characteristic of the flat bones of the cranial vault.

Meningocele Neural tube defect in which a sac of fluid-filled meninges protrudes through an opening in the skull or vertebrae

Mesencephalon One of the three primary brain vesicles that does not subdivide

Mesenchyme Any loosely organized tissue comprised of fibroblast-like cells and extracellular matrix, regardless of the origin of the cells

Mesentery Double layer of peritoneum that connects portions of the gut or other viscera to the body wall or to each other. Mesenteries provide pathways for nerves, blood vessels, and lymphatics to and from the viscera and help to support the organs in the abdomen.

Mesoderm One of three basic germ layers that forms blood vessels, bone, connective tissue, and other structures.

Mesonephros Primitive kidney that forms tubules and ducts in the thoracic and lumbar regions. Most of these structures degenerate, but the main duct (mesonephric duct) and some of the tubules contribute to the male reproductive system.

Mesonephric ducts Collecting ducts for the mesonephric kidney that regress in females, but form the epididymis, ductus deferens, seminal vesicle, and ejaculatory ducts in males

Metanephros Definitive kidney formed from metanephric mesoderm (metanephric blastema) in the pelvic region

Metencephalon Derived from the cranial portion of the rhombencephalon (hindbrain); forms the cerebellum and pons

Midgut Part of the gut tube extending from immediately distal to the liver bud to the proximal two thirds of the transverse colon. It forms part of the duodenum, jejunum, ileum, cecum, appendix, ascending colon, and part of the transverse colon. Early in development, it forms the primary intestinal loop with the superior mesenteric artery as its axis. This loop is involved in gut rotation and physiological umbilical herniation and is connected to the yolk sac by the vitelline duct.

Monozygotic twins Twins formed from a single oocyte. Splitting may occur at the two-cell stage or after formation of the germ disc, but usually takes place at the time of inner cell mass formation.

Morphogen Molecule secreted at a distance that can induce cells to differentiate. The same morphogen can induce more than one cell type by establishing a concentration gradient.

Müllerian-inhibiting substance Another term for the antimüllerian hormone that is produced by Sertoli cells and causes regression of the müllerian (paramesonephric) ducts in males

Myelencephalon Derived from the caudal portion of the rhombencephalon (hindbrain); forms the medulla oblongata

Myotome Dorsomedial portion of each somite that forms the epimere from which extensor muscles of the back are derived

Nephron Functional unit of the kidney consisting of the proximal and distal convoluted tubules, loop of Henle, Bowman's capsule, and a glomerulus

Neural crest cells Cells of the neuroepithelium that form at the tips ("crest") of the neural folds and then migrate to other regions to form many structures, including spinal ganglia, bones and connective tissue of the face, septa for the outflow tract of the heart, some cranial nerve ganglia, ganglia for the gut tube (enteric ganglia), melanocytes, and so on. These cells are vulnerable to teratogenic insult, explaining why many children with facial clefts also have cardiac defects.

Neurocranium Part of the skull that forms a protective case around the brain (the other part of the skull is the viscerocranium, or face). It consists of two parts, the membranous neurocranium or flat bones of the skull and the cartilaginous neurocranium or chondrocranium forming the base of the skull.

Neuropores Cranial and caudal openings of the developing neural tube, present from the time that the neural folds first make contact until the neural tube is complete, i.e., unclosed portions of the closing neural tube

Neurulation The process of transforming the neural plate into the neural tube. Neurulation begins in the 3rd week and ends at 28 days. Failure of the neural folds to close the tube results in neural tube defects, including anencephaly and spina bifida.

Notochord An extended column of midline cells lying immediately ventral to the floor plate of the central nervous system and extending from the hypophysis to the end of the spinal cord. It is important for inducing the neural plate, ventral (motor) region of the brain and spinal cord, and the sclerotome portion of the somites to form vertebrae. The major signal molecule for these phenomena is sonic hedgehog (SHH).

Nucleus pulposus Central gelatinous portion of an intervertebral disc derived from proliferation of notochord cells

Omentum Fold of peritoneum passing from the stomach to the liver (lesser omentum) or from the stomach to the transverse colon and beyond (greater omentum).

Outer cell mass Cells that surround the blastocyst cavity and cover the inner cell mass and that will form the trophoblast

Organogenesis Period of development when the organ primordia are established, usually considered to be from the beginning of the 3rd week to the end of the 8th week of gestation. This is the time when organs are most sensitive to insult and induction of most birth defects occurs.

Paramesonephric ducts Ducts that parallel the mesonephric duct and extend from the abdominal cavity to the posterior wall of the urogenital sinus. These ducts regress in the male, but form the uterus, uterine (fallopian) tubes, and upper part of the vagina in females.

Paraxial mesoderm Mesoderm-derived tissue along the axis of the embryo responsible for forming somites and somitomeres

Parenchyma The distinguishing cells of a gland or organ held together by connective tissue called the stroma

Parietal Pertaining to the wall of any cavity

Parturition Birth

Pericardioperitoneal canals Openings from the abdomen to the thorax posterior to the septum transversum that are closed by the pleuroperitoneal membranes during formation of the diaphragm

Pharyngeal arches Bars of mesenchyme derived from mesoderm and neural crest cells that form in five pairs

around the pharynx, somewhat like the gills (branchia) of a fish. They are covered by ectoderm externally and endoderm internally. Clefts are present externally between pairs of arches; pouches are present between arches internally. However, there is no communication between clefts and pouches.

Pharyngeal cleft Ectoderm-lined indentation between pharyngeal arches on their external surface

Pharyngeal pouch Endoderm-lined indentation between pharyngeal arches on their internal surfaces

Phenotype The physical characteristics of an individual

Placode A thickened region of ectoderm that forms sensory organs and ganglia. Examples include the nasal, otic, lens, and epibranchial placodes.

Pleuropericardial folds Extensions of mesoderm from the lateral body wall that meet in the midline to separate the pleural and pericardial cavities. The folds carry the phrenic nerve with them and contribute to the parietal pericardium and form the fibrous pericardium.

Pleuroperitoneal folds Extensions of mesoderm that extend from the body wall to meet the septum transversum and mesentery of the esophagus, thereby closing the pericardio-peritoneal canals during formation of the diaphragm.

Prechordal plate Collection of mesoderm cells lying between the bucco-pharyngeal membrane and the cranial end of the notochord. These cells represent some of the first to pass through the primitive streak and are important for forebrain induction using sonic hedgehog as a signal molecule.

Primary intestinal loop Loop formed around the superior mesenteric artery by the midgut. It rotates and lengthens as it herniates into the umbilicus in the 6th week. It then continues its growth and rotation as it re-enters the abdominal cavity beginning in the 10th week.

Primary palate Formed by the medial nasal prominences as part of the intermaxillary segment. It fuses with the secondary palate.

Primitive node Elevated region around the cranial end of the primitive streak that is known as the "organizer" because it regulates important processes such as laterality and formation of the notochord

Primitive pit Depression in the primitive node

Primitive streak Groove formed in the epiblast at the caudal end of the bilaminar germ disc stage embryo through which epiblast cells migrate to form endoderm and mesoderm during gastrulation

Processus vaginalis Outpocketing of peritoneum that precedes the testis through the inguinal canal. Once it reaches the scrotum, it pinches off from the abdominal cavity and forms the tunica vaginalis of the testis. If it fails to pinch off, it can serve as a path for herniation of bowel through the canal into the scrotum forming an inguinal (indirect) hernia.

Pronephros Primitive kidney that forms a few nonfunctional vestigial tubules in the cervical region

Prosencephalon One of three primary brain vesicles that forms the telencephalon and diencephalon

Rathke's pouch Outpocketing of ectoderm from the roof of the oral cavity that forms the anterior portion (adenohypophysis) of the pituitary

Rectouterine pouch (Douglas' pouch) Depression between the vagina and rectum. This site is the most common place for an ectopic pregnancy within the peritoneal cavity. (The most common site for ectopic pregnancies in general is in the ampullary region of the uterine tube).

Renal corpuscle Combination of Bowman's capsule and a glomerulus

Retroperitoneal Posterior to the peritoneum

Rhombencephalon One of three primary brain vesicles that forms the metencephalon and myelencephalon

Rhombomere One of eight segments that form in the rhombencephalon that contribute to development of cranial nerve nuclei and give rise to neural crest cells that migrate to the pharyngeal arches

Secondary palate Derived from the maxillary processes of the first arch; includes the soft and hard palates. Fuses with the primary palate anteriorly.

Sclerotome Ventromedial part of each somite that forms the vertebrae

Septum primum The first septum to grow down from the roof of the common atrium and contribute to the interatrial septum. Prior to contact with the atrioventricular endocardial cushions, programmed cell death creates a new opening in this septum to maintain communication between the atrial chambers. This septum forms the valve of the foramen ovale.

Septum secundum The second septum to grow down from the roof of the common atrium toward the atrioventricular endocardial cushions. It never makes contact with the cushions; consequently, an oblique opening, the foramen ovale, is created between the septum secundum and septum primum that allows shunting of blood from the right atrium to the left during fetal development. At birth, this opening is closed when the septum primum is pressed against the septum secundum and the adult pattern of blood flow is established.

Septum transversum Mesoderm tissue originally lying cranial to the heart, but repositioned between the heart and connecting stalk by cranial folding of the embryo. It gives rise to the central tendon of the diaphragm, connective tissue for the liver, and ventral mesentery.

Situs inversus Complete reversal of left- and right-sidedness of the organs in the thorax and abdomen

Somites Epithelial balls of cells formed in segmental pairs along the neural tube from paraxial mesoderm. Somites differentiate into vertebrae, muscles of the back and body wall, and dermis of the skin.

Somitomeres Loosely organized segmented collections of paraxial mesoderm in the cranial region. Somitomeres form muscles and bone of the face and skull.

Sonic hedgehog Secreted protein that acts as a morphogen in several embryonic sites, including the limbs, somites, gut formation, and establishment of the midline in the central nervous system

Spina bifida Neural tube defect that involves incomplete development of the vertebral arches, with or without defects of the underlying neural tube. If only the vertebrae are involved the defect is called spina bifida occulta, because it usually is skin-covered and not visible from the surface. If the underlying neural tube is affected, then the defect is called spina bifida cystica. Seventy percent of these defects can be prevented by daily maternal use of 400 μg of folic acid beginning 2 to 3 months prior to conception and continuing throughout pregnancy.

Spinal nerve Nerve formed by the junction of dorsal and ventral roots at each intervertebral foramen

Splanchnic nerves Preganglionic sympathetic and parasympathetic fibers in the thorax (greater [T5–9], lesser [T10 and 11], and least [T12] splanchnic nerves; sympathetic); lumbar region (lumbar splanchnics [L1 and 2]; sympathetic); and pelvic splanchnics (S2–4; parasympathetic).

Stenosis A narrowing of a canal or orifice

Stroma Connective tissue of glands

Surfactant Phospholipid made by alveolar type II cells that reduces surface tension in alveoli, a step that is essential for respiration. Production does not begin until the end of the 6th month, making it difficult for premature infants born before this time to survive.

Sympathetic trunks Paired collections of sympathetic ganglia lying on the posterior body wall lateral to the vertebral bodies; sometimes called sympathetic chain ganglia

Syncytiotrophoblast Outer multinucleated layer of the trophoblast that serves to invade the endometrium of the uterus

Syndrome A group of abnormalities occurring together that have a known cause, e.g., Down syndrome, fetal alcohol syndrome

Telencephalon Derived from the most cranial portion of the prosencephalon (forebrain); forms the cerebral hemispheres.

Teratogen A factor that causes a birth defect, such as a drug or environmental toxicant

Teratology Science that studies the origin, causes, and prevention of birth defects

Teratoma Tumor containing derivatives from all three germ layers. They may arise from remnants of the primitive streak or from germ cells that do not migrate successfully to the gonadal ridges. The most common ones are caudal teratomas arising in the buttock region.

Thyroglossal duct Duct formed along the path of thyroid migration extending in the midline from the foramen cecum in the tongue to the neck

Transcription factors Proteins with DNA binding sites that regulate expression of downstream genes

Trophoblast Outer cell layer surrounding the blastocyst from which placental tissues are derived

Urachus Vestigial remnant of the allantois from the ventral surface of the urogenital sinus to the umbilicus that normally regresses to a fibrous cord forming the median umbilical ligament. Sometimes it may remain patent to form an urachal fistula or cyst.

Urogenital ridge Bilateral epithelial-covered elevation of intermediate mesoderm that lies in the lower thoracic and lumbar regions and that forms the mesonephric kidneys and the gonads

Urorectal septum Wedge of mesoderm that grows down between the hindgut and primitive urogenital sinus, partially separating these two structures. The caudal end of the septum forms the perineal body.

Uterovesical pouch Depression between the vagina and the bladder

Ventral mesentery Double layer of peritoneum derived from the septum transversum and extending from the liver to the ventral body wall (the falciform ligament) and from the liver to the stomach and duodenum (lesser omentum).

Ventral primary ramus Ventral branch of a spinal nerve that innervates muscles derived from the hypomere and skin over the anterior body wall and limbs

Ventral root Motor fibers passing from ventral horn cells in the spinal cord to a spinal nerve

Visceral Relating to the organs of the body

Viscerocranium Part of the skull that comprises the bones of the face. (The other part of the skull is the neurocranium.)

Vitelline duct Connection between the yolk sac and the primary intestinal loop of the midgut through the connecting stalk. Failure of this duct to degenerate results in fistulas and diverticula (e.g., Meckel's diverticulum)

from the small intestine to the umbilicus.

White rami communicantes Connections carrying preganglionic sympathetic fibers from spinal nerves to the sympathetic trunks. White rami exist only at levels T1–L2.

Yolk sac Structure located ventral to the bilaminar germ disc derived from the hypoblast. It is the site of origin of the first blood cells and the germ cells and remains attached to the midgut via the vitelline (yolk sac) duct until late in development.

Zone of polarizing activity (ZPA) Population of mesoderm cells at the posterior border of the limb next to the apical ectodermal ridge that regulates anterior–posterior patterning of the limb

FIGURE CREDITS: ESSENTIAL LANGMAN

Figure 1.2A&B. Modified from Gilbert SF. *Developmental Biology.* Sunderland, MA: Sinaver, 2000.

Figure 2.1B&C. Courtesy of Dr. Caroline Ziomeck, Genzyme Transgenics Corporation.

Figure 2.3A. Modified from Hamilton WJ, Mossman HW. *Human Embryology.* Baltimore: Williams & Wilkins, 1972.

Figure 2.5B. Reprinted with permission from Smith JL, Gestland KM, Schoenwolf GC. Prospective fate map of the mouse primitive streak at 7.5 days of gestation. *Developmental Dynamics* 201:279, 1994.

Figure 2.5E. Courtesy Dr. K.K. Sulik, Department of Cell and Developmental Biology, University of North Carolina

Figure 2.8A. Courtesy of Dr. Don Nakayama, Department of Surgery, University of North Carolina

Figure 3.3. Courtesy Dr. K.K. Sulik, Department of Cell and Developmental Biology, University of North Carolina

Figure 3.4D. Courtesy Dr. K.K. Sulik, Department of Cell and Developmental Biology, University of North Carolina

Figure 3.9B. Reprinted with permission from Coletta PL, Shimeld SM, Sharpe P. The molecular anatomy of *Hox* gene expression. *Journal of Anatomy* 184:15, 1994.

Figure 3.10A. Courtesy of Dr. J. Warkany. Reprinted with permission from Warkany J. *Congenital Malformations.* Chicago, IL: Year Book Medical Publishers, 1971.

Figure 3.10B. Courtesy of Dr. M. J. Sellers, Division of Medical and Molecular Genetics, Guys Hospital, London.

Figure 3.11A. Courtesy of Dr. S. Lacey, Department of Surgery, University of North Carolina.

Figure 3.11B. Courtesy of Dr. S. Lacey, Department of Surgery, University of North Carolina.

Figure 4.1B. Modified from Gilbert SF. *Developmental Biology.* Sunderland, MA: Sinaver, 2000.

Figure 4.2. Reprinted with permission from Heuser CH. A presomite embryo with a definite chorda canal. *Contributions in Embryology* 23:253, 1932. Courtesy of Carnegie Institution of Washington, Washington, DC.

Figure 4.3A. Modified from Noden DM. Interactions and fates of avarian craniofacial mesenchyme. *Development* 103:121–140, 1988.

Figure 4.4C-F. Reprinted with permission from Muenke M, Schell U. Fibroblast growth factor receptor mutations in human skeletal disorders. *Trends in Genetics* 2:308–313, 1995.

Figure 4.5E. Larsen WJ. *Human Embryology.* 4th ed. New York, NY: Churchill Livingston, 2001

Figure 4.6A-C. Courtesy Dr. K.K. Sulik, Department of Cell and Developmental Biology, University of North Carolina

Figure 4.6G-J. Modified from Gilbert SF. *Developmental Biology.* Sunderland, MA: Sinaver, 2000.

Figure 4.7A-H. Shubin N, Tabin C, Carroll S. Fossils, genes and the evolution of animal limbs. *Nature* 388:639–648, 1997.

Figure 4.8C. Reprinted with permission from Stevenson RE, Hall JG, Goodman RM (eds). *Human Malformations and Related Anomalies.* New York, NY: Oxford University Press, 1993.

Figure 4.9. From Moore & Dalley, COA, LWW, 4th ed.

Figure 4.11. Courtesy of Dr. D. Nakayama, Department of Surgery, University of North Carolina

Figure 5.1H-J. Modified from Marvin MJ, di Rocco J, Gardiner A, Bush SM, Lassar AB. Inhibition of Wnt activity induces heart formation from posterior mesoderm. *Genes in Development* 15:316, 2001.

Figure 5.2E, 5.3F&G, 5.6A, 5.7D&I. Courtesy Dr. K.K. Sulik, Department of Cell and Developmental Biology, University of North Carolina

Figure 6.3E. Modified from Gilbert SF. *Developmental Biology.* Sunderland, MA: Sinaver, 2000.

Figure 6.5P. From Moore & Dalley, COA, LWW, 4th ed.

Figure 6.6D. Courtesy Dr. K.K. Sulik, Department of Cell and Developmental Biology, University of North Carolina

Figure 6.8B&E. Reprinted with permission from Nievelstein RAJ, Van Der Werff JFA, Verbeek FJ, Valk J, Verneij-Keers C. Normal and abnormal embryonic development of the anorectum in human embryos. *Teratology* 57:70–78, 1998.

Figure 7.3F. Reprinted with permission from Stevenson RE, Hall JG, Goodman RM (eds). *Human Malformations and Related Anomalies.* New York, NY: Oxford University Press, 1993.

Figure 7.4A,D&E. Reprinted with permission from Stevenson RE, Hall JG, Goodman RM (eds). *Human Malformations and Related Anomalies.* New York, NY: Oxford University Press, 1993.

Figure 7.6G&H. Reprinted with permission from Stevenson RE, Hall JG, Goodman RM (eds). *Human Malformations and Related Anomalies.* New York, NY: Oxford University Press, 1993.

Figure 7.11C&H, 7.12C&D. Courtesy Dr. K.K. Sulik, Department of Cell and Developmental Biology, University of North Carolina

Figure 7.14. Courtesy of Dr. R.J. Gorlin, Department of Oral Pathology and Genetics, University of Minnesota.

Figure 8.1C&D. Courtesy Dr. K.K. Sulik, Department of Cell and Developmental Biology, University of North Carolina

Figure 8.3B. Reprinted with permission from Krumlauf R. Hox genes and pattern formation in the branchial region of the vertebrate head. *Trends in Genetics* 9:106–112, 1993.

Figure 8.5A. Courtesy of Dr. J. Warkany. Reprinted with permission from Warkany J. *Congenital Malformations.* Chicago, IL: Year Book Medical Publishers, 1971.

Figure 8.5B-D. Courtesy of Dr. R.J. Gorlin, Department of Oral Pathology and Genetics, University of Minnesota.

Figure 8.6C,F&H, 8.7A,D,E,H&K, 8.8A. Courtesy Dr. K.K. Sulik, Department of Cell and Developmental Biology, University of North Carolina

Figure 8.8E,G&I. Courtesy of Dr. M. Edgerton, Department of Plastic Surgery, University of Virginia.

Figure 8.8K,L&M. Courtesy of Dr. R.J. Gorlin, Department of Oral Pathology and Genetics, University of Minnesota.

Figure 8.9B&D, 9.1B,D&F, 9.3A-C. Courtesy Dr. K.K. Sulik, Department of Cell and Developmental Biology, University of North Carolina

Figure 9.7. Redrawn from Cordes SP. Molecular genetics of cranial nerve development in mouse. *Nat Rev Neurosci* 2:611–615, 2001.

Figure 9.8. Adapted from Noden DM. Interactions and fates of avian craniofacial mesenchyme. *Development* 103:121–140, 1988, Company of Biologists, Ltd.

Figure 9.9B. Moore & Dalley. COA, LWW, 4th ed.

Figure 9.10A-F. Redrawn from Tanabe Y, Jessell TM. Diversity and pattern in the developing spinal cord. *Science* 274:1115, 1996.

Figure 9.10G. Reprinted with permission from Krumlauf R. Hox genes and pattern formation in the branchial region of the vertebrate head. *Trends in Genetics* 9:106–112, 1993.

Figure 9.10I. Redrawn from Lumsden A, Krumlauf R. Patterning the vertebrate axis. *Science* 112:1109–1114, 1996.

Figure 9.11B. Courtesy of Dr. R.J. Gorlin, Department of Oral Pathology and Genetics, University of Minnesota.

Figure 9.11D. Courtesy of Dr. R.J. Gorlin, Department of Oral Pathology and Genetics, University of Minnesota.

Figure 10.1D,E,J&K. Courtesy Dr. K.K. Sulik, Department of Cell and Developmental Biology, University of North Carolina

Figure 10.3. Modified from Ashery-Padan R, Gruss P. Pax6 lights up the way for eye development. *Current Opinion in Cell Biology* 13:706, 2001.

Figure 10.4A,D,G,H&I. Courtesy Dr. K.K. Sulik, Department of Cell and Developmental Biology, University of North Carolina.

Figure 10.6G. Reprinted with permission from Moore KL. *Clinically Oriented Anatomy.* Baltimore: Williams & Wilkins, 1992:764.

Figure 10.7B&C. Courtesy Dr. K.K. Sulik, Department of Cell and Developmental Biology, University of North Carolina.

Figure 10.7G-J. Courtesy of Dr. R.J. Gorlin, Department of Oral Pathology and Genetics, University of Minnesota.

Figure 11.4F-I. Reprinted with permission from Stevenson RE, Hall, JG, Goodman RM (eds). *Human Malformations and Related Anomalies.* New York, NY: Oxford University Press, 1993.

Figure 11.6A-D,G&H. Courtesy of Dr. Hytham Imseis, Department of Obstetrics and Gynecology, Mountain Area Health Education Center, Asheville, NC.

Figure 11.6E&F. Courtesy of Dr. Nancy Chescheir, Department of Obstetrics and Gynecology, University of North Carolina.

INDEX

Page numbers followed by f denote figures; t, tables